# FOUR
# UMBRELLAS

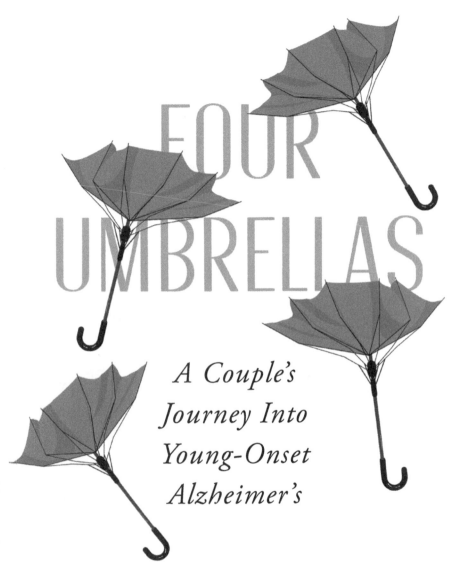

# FOUR UMBRELLAS

## *A Couple's Journey Into Young-Onset Alzheimer's*

### JUNE HUTTON & TONY WANLESS

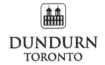

DUNDURN
TORONTO

Publisher: Scott Fraser | Acquiring editor: Kathryn Lane | Editor: Dominic Farrell
Cover designer: Laura Boyle
Cover image: shutterstock.com/ArtService
Printer: Marquis Book Printing Inc.

"Not Me" first published in *Other Voices* [1999/Volume 12, Number 1], © H. June Hutton.
A portion of the proceeds from the sale of *Four Umbrellas* will be donated by the authors to Paul's Club, paulsclub.weebly.com.

Library and Archives Canada Cataloguing in Publication

Title: Four umbrellas : a couple's journey into young-onset Alzheimer's / June Hutton & Tony Wanless.
Names: Hutton, June, 1954- author. | Wanless, Tony, 1949- author.
Identifiers: Canadiana (print) 20200281615 | Canadiana (ebook) 20200281623 | ISBN 9781459747791 (softcover) | ISBN 9781459747807 (PDF) | ISBN 9781459747814 (EPUB)
Subjects: LCSH: Wanless, Tony, 1949-—Health. | LCSH: Hutton, June, 1954-—Marriage. | LCSH: Alzheimer's disease—Patients—Biography. | LCSH: Alzheimer's disease—Patients—Family relationships. | LCSH: Spouses—Biography. | LCGFT: Autobiographies.
Classification: LCC RC523.2 .H88 2020 | DDC 362.1968/3110092—dc23

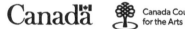   

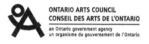 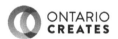

We acknowledge the support of the Canada Council for the Arts and the Ontario Arts Council for our publishing program. We also acknowledge the financial support of the Government of Ontario, through the Ontario Book Publishing Tax Credit and Ontario Creates, and the Government of Canada.

Care has been taken to trace the ownership of copyright material used in this book. The author and the publisher welcome any information enabling them to rectify any references or credits in subsequent editions.

The publisher is not responsible for websites or their content unless they are owned by the publisher.

Printed and bound in Canada.

VISIT US AT

 dundurn.com | 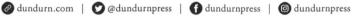 @dundurnpress |  dundurnpress |  dundurnpress

Dundurn
3 Church Street, Suite 500
Toronto, Ontario, Canada
M5E 1M2

*To the kids*
*who are no longer kids*
*may they never have to go through this*

# A TRAJECTORY OF CHANGE

His shoulder bag is open on the floor. On his knees and still in his stocking feet, he roots through it, calling out to me that he can't find his keys. He upends the black bag and pulls out a hat, gloves, an umbrella, and a plastic bread bag.

The bread bag is plucked up next, and out tumbles his phone, wallet, notebook, and pen — all kept in the plastic bag so they won't get wet if it rains. But still no keys.

Now he's pulling open the cupboard drawers, rifling through them, yanking coats from hangers in the open closet to search the pockets. Next, the laundry bag.

A pile of clothes and possessions is growing on the floor of his home office that he fastidiously tidied yesterday, a task that took him all day.

You don't need your keys, I assure him. We can use mine.

He shouts at me to stop shouting at him.

I blink. Perhaps I had been. I try again: We're going to be late.

Grudgingly, he stops the search, sits on a chair and slips on his shoes, ties the laces. Painfully slowly, it seems to me, he stuffs his wallet and phone and notebook into the plastic bread bag and puts it back into his shoulder bag. I know better than to offer to help.

There is no time to tidy up the room and I hold my breath as he stands, worried that he will insist.

He starts to bend and I remind him: We're getting the answers today. We'd better hurry.

To my relief, he straightens, puts on his coat and hat.

We are about to head out the front door when, in a burst of inspiration, he darts over to the hallway closet to yank open those doors and emerges, triumphant, brandishing the missing keys.

Then he asks me, Where are we going, again?

We hurry outside, clutching our collars against the gusts of wind.


Spring is a fickle time of year: soft and scented one day, raw and cold the next. The season's very unpredictability makes it an especially suitable time to start this narrative, one that is full of delays and disappointments, conflicting evidence and opinions, as well as, occasionally, periods of peace along with misplaced contentment — all of them swirling around us, rising and settling and then rising again. All because no one could tell us what was wrong, could even acknowledge that anything was wrong.

Waiting has been, at times, unbearable. The process of getting a diagnosis dragged on for more than just one season; it lasted several years. It's April 2018 now, and as we head to the hospital again, we fear that the final answer to our question of what is wrong will be devastating.

At the centre of this story is one of the smartest people I know, a journalist named Tony Wanless.

Many of us claim to be better in one area of learning than another, at reading and writing, for instance, than at math and science, or vice versa. You can see my own bias in the way I ordered that sentence. Tony, however, was one of those rare individuals who was accomplished in both areas. He excelled in Latin and algebra, in science and the arts; he skipped a grade in high school. He had the sort of mind that easily grasped foreign languages, a skill due in part to the fact that he was born in the Netherlands where his family spoke Dutch. He was a toddler when they moved to Canada, and while he studied French at school, it was English that became the language used at home. His facility with language would become his greatest strength, leading him away from studies in engineering to a career in journalism.

Despite his talent and accomplishments, he has suffered from depression all his life. Perhaps, given his difficult family history, this isn't so surprising. Tony says his father had a temper and, within a couple of years of their arrival, unhappy to be working in Dutch farming communities in Ontario, he hatched a plan to rob a credit union. Tony's mother worked nights as a cleaner for the credit union, and he wanted her to let him in. She refused and threatened to expose him. He beat her unconscious in front of the children, and he was subsequently deported, not for the beating, but for the planned robbery. She raised three children on her own, which couldn't have been easy. When she remarried, to a Chatham resident of British background named Lyle Wanless, Tony traded his long Dutch birth name, Antonius

Josefus Franciscus Stephanos Maria Versteeg, for an English one: Tony Wanless.

Just after he left his studies in engineering, Tony returned to the Netherlands. It was his first trip back since he'd emigrated in early childhood. He looked up his father, who he hadn't seen since the deportation. Tony found him in a welfare lineup, a broken-down man, older than his years, who lived on a canal barge with a large dog. It could have been a sad or angry meeting, and yet old Willem Versteeg paraded his son about the neighbourhood, clearly proud and happy in that moment, and in the end, so was Tony.

While Tony has had his dark moments, he can be very upbeat, and throughout his life he has made friends easily. Holland was a great adventure. He entered a contest to see who could roll the largest joint, and won, his prize being said enormous joint. He also auditioned for the musical *Hair*, infamous for its nude scene, thinking his willingness to step onto the stage naked would surely get him the part, only to discover they were seeking singing talent as well.

When he returned home, he enrolled in a federal government work program in journalism. His sheer enthusiasm for life, his love of talking — oh, how he talks — combined with his smarts, made this an ideal career choice. He never looked back.

Tony worked at various newspapers, from the *Windsor Star*, the *Toronto Sun*, and the *Brampton Times*, to the *Calgary Herald*, before finally heading to the West Coast. A likable guy, Tony had his share of girlfriends, but he had never married. We met on the rewrite desk in the Pacific Press newsroom in Vancouver. The first thing I noticed about him were his large, tanned hands — farmer's hands, he called them — typing adeptly on the keyboard. I was immediately smitten by his looks — his curly hair and big blue eyes — but I was wary. I was in the process of a divorce. It was too soon. I was also a single mother who had her child's feelings to consider, and that made Tony wary, too. He played hard to get.

We did, at last, start dating. He began making moves toward a committed relationship, but it was slow going. We danced around the subject for a year, eventually buying a townhouse and moving in together. Tony said that for him, a financial commitment was more binding than a ring. I had been married, and while I knew that wasn't the answer to everything, I also knew avoidance when I heard it.

Then my son, Garth, became gravely ill with the HSP (Henoch-Schönlein purpura) virus, often triggered in children by another illness, in his case, strep throat. He recovered, but during the height of the illness, Tony took on a full caring role, from staying up nights to sharing shifts with me at the hospital, and my child became our child. Tony often comments that the thing he is most proud of is raising Garth. Somewhere back in those days of shared parenting, when Tony finally made the leap and became, in the fullest sense, my partner, we found the kind of love that made commitment a natural next step.

He was ready to get married. I admit I was somewhat exasperated by the timing. Months before, when the subject first came up, I had been all for it. This time, I was training for a new career in teaching, and had already extended my practicum to allow for the time away to look after Garth when he'd been ill. If Tony wanted a wedding, I told him that he'd have to plan it himself. I wasn't being nasty. I simply didn't have time. To my surprise, he did it. Perhaps turning forty had had an effect on him, but he got going and arranged a beautiful open-air wedding at the Beach House in Stanley Park.

We were comfortable in each other's company and became good friends. Did we ever argue? You bet. Heatedly. However, he was the first person I would talk to if something went well, or didn't. If I had a creative idea, I couldn't wait to get home and share it. Our love of news and writing was a binding force. We didn't go everywhere together as some couples do. We had our own areas of interest, even within writing — his, business, mine, literary — and even at the same parties we would move about independently, re-convening now and then, until it was time to go home. And then we would talk all the way back, sharing what we had experienced.

The only time I saw evidence of depression in Tony, initially, was over money. He liked to save, and parting with money always caused him great grief. This raised many jokes at work. Even his mother would poke fun, calling him "a cheap Dutchman." He was able to laugh at himself, though, and undertook a news column that he titled "The Cheap Guy."

During the first years of our married life, I would call out questions to Tony, such as, How do you spell this? Or, Who ran the country during the Forties? Or, When were antibiotics discovered? This was lazy of me, I admit. My reasoning, however, was simple: Why should I look things up when I knew he would have the answers right there in his head? Tony read voraciously; he soaked up words and information.

When did all that change? Certainly, there is no denying that it did.

On that spring day in 2018, we arrive, and just in time, at the Djavad Mowafaghian Centre for Brain Health at the University of British Columbia hospital in Vancouver.

We approach the building with its magnificent windows of etched glass, patterns of brain cells that look astonishingly like the tentacles of an octopus, and Tony asks me again, What are we here for?

I repeat what I had said at home as well as on the way over, that we are here to see the neurologist, and to get the test results.

Have I met him before?

I assure him we both have, and Tony nods.

We have a good idea what this neurologist will tell us. Even so, we need to hear it from him.

It shouldn't have taken so long.

From as early as 2011, Tony had been growing increasingly forgetful and confused. The bright mind that had skipped a grade and excelled at Latin and algebra was failing him.

He had a fall, and I suspected a stroke. There were computed tomography (CT) scans and other scans, all showing nothing. There were doctors' appointments and memory tests, such as the Montreal Cognitive Assessment (MoCA), often with long stretches of time between them, which had led to the observation that he had mild cognitive impairment, or MCI.

MCI is often called a holding-pattern diagnosis, because it is a condition that can remain stable, can even improve, or can worsen. Time, we were told, would determine the outcome.

Tony set his sights on improvement and, as he would, read everything he could find on the brain. He worked hard, and often scored high on the MoCA. The assessment is comprised of simple tests that take about ten minutes and require the person to do such tasks as memorize five words, draw a clock face to show a certain time, and answer questions about current events. He once surprised his gerontologist with a near-perfect total of twenty-eight out of thirty. Scores of twenty-six and higher are considered normal.

Over time, though, Tony's condition worsened, despite the prescription in 2015 of a drug called Aricept, to help improve his cognitive function. Had he had a stroke, after all? Or was it something else? There was the nagging question that had always been there, way in the back of my mind: Did he have dementia? I knew what the signs looked like. My mother had been diagnosed with Alzheimer's several years before and had been prescribed the same medication.

So was it actually Alzheimer's? The terms *possible*, *probable*, and *all indications are* were offered to us; they swirled about us in a cloud of vague potential outcomes. At the same time as we struggled to find an answer to what was wrong, we, and especially I, endured the frustration of having friends, family, and casual observers comment that Tony seemed just fine.

We pushed to see a neurologist, hoping for a magnetic resonance imaging (MRI) scan and a definitive diagnosis. Eventually, in the spring of 2017, we got the appointment. Again, Tony's MoCA score was not bad — twenty-six out of thirty. Further tests would be needed. After all, it could be normal aging.

I was appalled to hear that. I had seen this before and there was nothing normal about it. Tony himself was growing concerned. Did no one believe us?

Finally, six months later, Tony received the MRI, though we would have to wait another six months, until January of 2018, for a day-long series of neuropsychological memory tests before we could get the combined results — something that we would receive several more months after that.

Now, at last, in April of 2018, we are getting those combined results.

The Centre for Brain Health is home to UBC Hospital's Alzheimer's Clinic. As we pass through the doors, my eyes flick toward the sign and then back. Tony doesn't remark. A doctor assisting the neurologist is there. Tony is given the MoCA again and is asked a few questions. I am asked a few questions as well, mostly about his memory. We then settle into chairs in the examination room, and wait. The neurologist appears and sits down with us to tell us that the MRI showed atrophy, or shrinkage, in the temporal lobe areas of the brain, as well as evidence of small vessel disease, or mini-strokes. Whether these mini-strokes had caused Tony's fall in 2011 he can't say, but in the end he stresses that it is the series of neuropsychological tests that are particularly telling.

In every category, Tony had done fairly well, except memory.

As the doctor talks, I recall movies and anecdotal accounts of the brilliant scientist who could still calculate intricate formulas but could not remember the day of the week or the time of year. In the documentary *Spirit Unforgettable*, John Mann, lead singer of the band Spirit of the West and an Alzheimer's sufferer, scored eighteen on the MoCA test. A neurologist interviewed in the film said words to the effect that a score that low leaves no doubt: That's Alzheimer's.

Right on cue, this doctor confirms that the tests plus the results of the MRI show that Tony is in the early stages of Alzheimer's disease. He notes the positive effects of the drug Aricept on Tony's memory, and says that in Tony's case the progress of the disease is relatively slow but, even so, he had noticed a decline over the past year.

This doesn't sink in until I see the new MoCA results. The score this time is just twenty out of thirty.

I stand up to thank the doctor, and stagger as though drunk.

We finally have our answer, and a firm one. The words *probable* and *possible* that we had been hearing all this time have vanished.

We step out into the sunshine; the air is fresh and cool. The blustery spring weather is no surprise in April, and yet it seems a cruel trick somehow, so full of promise, of renewal.

Tony turns to the left and I reach for his elbow and turn him to the right, to the bus stop.

We will go home and I will feed the cats and make dinner and he will fall asleep somewhere along the way, exhausted. Nothing has changed and yet everything has.

That's a cliché, I know. It's a good one.

People often ask me, How did you know? What were the first signs? They are taking note, making comparisons, examining themselves or others close to them. Statistics show that the number of people diagnosed with Alzheimer's disease and other dementias increases every year, and still the cause is unknown.

Sometimes the signs are right there, if you know what to look for. Other times, they are only recognizable in retrospect. This is particularly the case with people like Tony, who show symptoms when they are under the age of sixty-five.

Many of us think of Alzheimer's as something our relatives might get in their eighties. We don't expect that a type of Alzheimer's called *early-* or *young-onset* could strike our family members, co-workers, or peers, two, three, sometimes even four, decades earlier.

It took seven years for us to get a final diagnosis, but, in fact, I had been seeing indications long before Tony's fall in 2011. The fall just provided something concrete, something to point to and examine.

In early 2017, we decided to write a book about the experience. There was nothing we could do about the outcome, but we hoped that if we wrote down what we had gone through, something could be learned. We decided to use email as a method of corresponding back and forth. This was a place to answer those questions, note down those first signs, those gut reactions, those fears.

No two people remember the same incident the same way, of course, and we all forget things. However, Tony's memory is especially susceptible to gaps. So, a record of this sort raises the whole issue of reliability. Even in the process of recalling, we are questioning the nature of memory, the hazy lens through which we examine our pasts.

My role is particularly troubling. Am I the conduit through which Tony tells his story? This book as a whole could not have been created if it were left to him to write. He can no longer manage the intricacies of structure and the organizing of details, so it has fallen on me to devise the framework and write the narrative. There have been decisions I've had to make on my own: how to deal with dates, which I've had to sort out and order as best they can be, given the accessibility of records and information; which facts and statistics to incorporate given the huge number available to choose from; and, most importantly, how much to include, how much to leave out. This is a shared journey in which I am also the caregiver, and yet repeatedly I wonder: Is there too much me in this story? I will grapple with all this and more throughout the telling.

In one of his earliest emails to me in 2017, Tony still refused to believe, despite mounting evidence, that he had dementia, though he was acutely aware that something was wrong. In the following note, as with the other written contributions from him, the errors, gaps, and repetitions, along with parenthetical comments, are tangible evidence of the disease's impact, and are left as is for that reason.

> It's been slightly more than a year since I was diagnosed with MCI.
>
> I was becoming increasingly forgetful. More important and frightening to me, however, was that it was becoming increasingly more difficult to focus. I would get bored and drift away while doing something, whether talking with someone, or involved with something that I found tedious, then suddenly "wake up" and remember where I was and "get back to work." It was as if my mind became un-anchored and just bobbed along in the water drifting with the current for a bit – a nice, stress-free feeling, by the way. This also meant it became increasingly difficult

to work, which meant I was constantly looking for distraction, i.e., computer, talking with Husein, who shared the office with me and eventually stopped coming in). Of course, this also led to depression (which probably increased the problem) because business and many other things were failing.

My research tells me this is common with MCI (although it has to be gleaned from all the chaff about Alzheimer's, which rarely seems relevan, I guess because more complete brain breakdown is "sexier" for most researchers and writers.

Later, Tony would add:

MCI is a lessening of some mental abilities like memory, impulse control and cognition (i.e. word recall, mathematics, handwriting, etc). It's a condition that's on the Alzheimer's scale, although it doesn't necessarily develop into Alzheimers (about a 30% chance, I was told. Regarding the other 70%, the condition remains the same or reverses).

Understandably, the absence of a definitive diagnosis had allowed him to form a half-truth, in which all he was suffering from was this thing called MCI, and that he could beat it.

We are writers, and it is only natural we would head to our keyboards to sort out our thoughts. This last correspondence might also prove a final comfort, not only for Tony and me but for others reading our story. In these pages, we are comparing notes, yet at the same time we are also reaching out, wondering who else might be reading this and looking for answers, too.

# PART ONE

# LOOKING BACK

# EARLY WARNING SIGNS

I n 1996, we were living in an old house near the graveyard. The proximity didn't concern us. Mountain View is a mature cemetery with large trees, and our dog Katie enjoyed long walks over the rolling hills.

The house had been our friend Terri's place, one that had been rented for several years after she and her family moved from Vancouver to New York City. When we bought it, we tore up the carpets that had protected the wood floors underneath. We had the boards lightly sanded, and then stained, and they took on a rich, golden tone. There were four bedrooms on the second level, which meant that in addition to our room and a guest room we each got an office, a luxury after nine years in a cramped townhouse. Garth got the attic room — a large rambling space.

We painted walls and bought vintage wooden wardrobes. The south-facing backyard was all lawn, but Tony went about planting a garden, and within a couple of years there were trees and shrubs and glorious shade. I set aside a patch for vegetables, but focused mostly on the front yard, planting daisies and foxglove and holly-hock — heritage blooms to match the old house.

Every February, I would find Tony at the back door, staring out at the yard, planning. His struggles with depression seemed to lessen when he was gardening.

He did the heavy-duty sort of yard work. No weeding for him; instead, he was out there digging trenches, uprooting and replant-ing the heavy rhodos, moving plants until they reached a pleas-ant symmetry — and then he'd start all over again the next year. He was keeping fit. He also rode his bike to work at the news-paper each day, a healthy habit he'd started when we lived in our townhouse near city hall. Those long rides to downtown probably helped lessen his dark moods, too.

We lived in that house for just seven years, but in that short time, things changed. At a certain point during this period, the gardening and the bike rides were no longer enough to chase away the darkness, and so Tony began to take anti-depressants.

After a while, he also began to neglect the garden. Not that it was a mess, but the plants stayed exactly where he'd put them. There was no more staring out at the backyard in February, planning.

I have photographs of my mother from that time, taken in the yard. She used to share his love of gardening, and he often sought her advice. But within a couple of years of us moving into the house, he said he noticed that her interest had faded and many of his ques-tions went unanswered. Eventually, he stopped asking them. She had been diagnosed with Alzheimer's disease, but I didn't make the leap from her loss of interest to his, even though they overlapped. Why would I? Tony was only fifty-two; she was twenty years older.

I felt I must have pushed him into something he'd never wanted. Maintaining the house had been a delightful challenge for him, but after a few years it seemed that he found it wearying, and the needed repairs were an aggravation. He wanted to sell the place.

And his job? It just wasn't what it used to be, he said. He began to talk of taking the severance package that Pacific Press was offering. That would give him three years' salary and a chance to run his own business. It was exactly what I had been talking about for myself for years: leaving my teaching job at an alternative school for at-risk youths so that I could write. He had always objected, so I was making the move gradually, going part-time, and writing on the side until several of my short stories and poems were published. I wondered if my small success — one literary magazine paid me all of $25 for a story called "Not Me" that took two years to write — had somehow encouraged him to make the leap. In 2002 he left the newsroom.

Encouraged in kind, I worked another year, watching his progress, and then I went on leave. Going on leave provided a safety net: I could return to work if it turned out I couldn't write something as challenging as a novel.

In 2003 we went to Spain. Tony had received the first third of his buyout payments, and his freelance work was earning him some money. I had saved up in preparation for my leave of absence. I needed the time to write, but I had also been helping to care for my mother. However, her health, though failing, had stabilized since she had been placed in a care home the year before. Why not go to Spain for a couple of weeks while we had the chance? The novel that I was working on required research in Spain, and Tony's nephew Dan was a jazz trumpeter in Barcelona.

It was a better trip than I could have imagined. The weather beautiful, the people friendly. Barcelona is a city of art and architecture — and music, thanks to Dan.

We ate delicious food and learned to appreciate cava, the Spanish sparkling wine. From Barcelona, we took a train through tunnels that bore into the mountains, revealing, when we emerged, in brilliant splashes of light between each peak, a turquoise ocean. In Tarragona, after viewing its Roman ruins, we set out again, this time by car, with Tony driving because I've never mastered standard shift, and in Spain, it seems, no one drives an automatic.

I would soon feel guilty about that.

We passed orchards and olive groves, stopping at the town of Belchite to view the preserved Civil War ruins for my research. From there, we headed to the Basque region and Pamplona, for fun.

We got caught up in the road system circling the town. It is neither a ring road nor a roundabout, but a series of curving roads connected by straight stretches — almost like the petals of a flower, only less even. We could see our destination, a little hotel near the famed bull ring, yet we could never find the exit road that would take us there. With each loop, Tony grew increasingly agitated. I was glad I wasn't driving.

And then I wished I was, because he not only refused to pull over and ask for directions, but his anger began to escalate. It seemed out of proportion to the problem — but why? I hadn't yet grasped the possible reason. He began shouting, swearing, and, most frightening of all, pressing down harder on the gas pedal and accelerating to speeds that took my breath away — and took us even farther from our destination.

Over and over and around and around again, Tony floored it, speeding through the streets of Pamplona. The only thing that stopped him was the sight of an armed guard.

We tell a funny story about this. The guard pulled his rifle from his shoulder and aimed it at the wild-eyed guy who burst out of his car door. Undaunted by the sight of weaponry, Tony ran across the road shouting, *Soy quarto Basquo!* I'm a quarter Basque! whereupon the guard re-shouldered his rifle, slapped Tony on the back like they were old Basque friends, and directed him to the right street.

Still, the manic drive that led to this moment returns to me often. Was that the beginning? Marital spats over driving and directions are the norm, aren't they? So why does this one stand out? I would have been too preoccupied in the moment to recall that just a couple of years previously, my mother had pounded my father's arm with her fist as he tried to navigate busy Kingsway in Vancouver after a snowfall. Driving in snow had always made her anxious, but the added impact of Alzheimer's disease turned this normally passive woman abusive. Ironically, it was her very actions that made the drive dangerous. That incident must have been hovering in my thoughts, producing a flutter of recognition, as I looked at Tony driving in Spain and saw something beyond road rage. I would see such behaviour many more times in the future. So, was that an early sign? Or was his decision to leave work a sign? Tony's job in journalism had been his whole life, his identity, and then, suddenly, he quit. And what of his passion for the house and garden? A few weeks after returning from Spain, we sold the place.

When I was building a narrative from our 2017 emails and showed Tony what I had written so far, I hoped he would respond, and expected he would place emphasis on different memories. After all, these events had happened many years before. In a sense, his response did just that, as there is no mention of Pamplona. But the last line had me lowering the page, and thinking, thinking.

Frankly, I had forgotten about much of this, although you painting a picture brought a lot of it back to mind. This is especially so with the house, and my enthusiasm, or later lack of it. I'm not sure why I lost enthusiasm for the house, but I suspected it had something to do with mid-life crisis.

Or not. Maybe it was simply that the rush of the new life was enough to stave off the usual depression for some time — ie, the thrill of a finally being a homeowner (without apostrophes, since my computer suddenly won't make them — something to do with the french, I think. I fixed it once before but can't remember how I did it so will have to figure it out again) ... had faded somewhat and it started to become a drag, a chore that just wasn't that exciting, or more likely seemed to be overwhelming.

I had always been better at bursts of energy and enthusiasm, and then becoming ... bored, I guess is the closest word, although that wasn't really true ... more like I was great at starting and working on things in shortish bursts but when I had to do the same thing again and again, grew impatient and depressed because it wasnèt so new — I was, I believe, a novelty junky — still am, I guess to a much lesser extent. It is as if I wanted to explore new territory, mostly with an overview rather than in depth. Thinking back on that, I was always like that. I think our marrying was the only time I was able to tear myself out of that mindset.

I think we might have even talked about it at the time, and I put it down to my regular depression — that could also have been the spring, when my usual winter blues were just peaking. I hadn't really realized at the time. But looking back at it, I realize it was just a revival of that old wandering spirit, although it wasn't anywhere nearly that romantic. It was more like constant searching — for what I don't know.

To circle all this back to the house and why we left it; I think some of it was because I needed change, and, as usual felt trapped. Whether all these changes happened in sequence or were just all jumbled up in my mind, Ièm not sure now. But I do know that the recurring pattern is excitement, boredom, desperation for something different, and eventually a leap into new and exciting. The key factor that worked itès way into this sequence, however, was that each time I was a older, more worn out from all the pressure and mental ups and downs. When I was in the newsroom, we used to talk about the "long, slow fade" that seemed to be the way of the world.

I believe now that I was starting it then.

# RESTLESS

When we look back, we peer through the lens of today. We form a theory of the past and then go searching for proof. It's why we yearn for a diagnosis, a name for what we are seeing. Without one, the symptoms lack definition, are only fearful suspicions that, like the nightmares of our childhoods, become something to dismiss. As children, we know with conviction that to reach the bedroom door we have to take a flying leap from the bed to avoid the snakes that live underneath. Same with that closet door. To open it at night when the lights are out ensures that a monster will jump out.

As adults, of course, we laugh at these memories.

At first, we might think the glitches and blips that form the early warning signs of Alzheimer's are the adult version of snakes under the bed. We tell ourselves they are not indicative of anything serious, but of course they are. The signs increase in number and intensity until we can't dismiss them any longer. They are leading to one clear conclusion. And we ask ourselves: Why didn't we notice any sooner?

We did. We just didn't know what it was we were seeing.

The medical experts we sought seemed, initially, equally unable to identify what was wrong. Doctors want to be absolutely certain before making a diagnosis that is life-altering — life-ending, in fact. I can't blame them for that, but I do blame them for not ordering the MRI and other tests that would have made it certain many years sooner.


There are times I don't want to write this book. Many people are unaware of Tony's disease. If we were to keep it that way, would the stress of it be easier to handle? Does coming out about Tony's Alzheimer's really help anyone?

The last thing I have ever wanted to write was a memoir. I call this narrative creative non-fiction, because otherwise, who do we think we are? Memoirs are written by famous people who've accomplished great things. And again, doesn't *memoir* invite the presence of too much me?

Questions upon questions. Am I revealing too much — or not enough? Am I holding back? Am I exaggerating the negative because it makes for better drama? I cringe at the very words I have written about Tony, his gaps, his blunders, his struggle to continue. Pamplona was a tough one to record. These are not criticisms of him, but notes of early signs of the disease.

If I were a scientist or medical professional, I might distinguish between the words *symptoms* and *signs*, the first being what is experienced by the person with Alzheimer's, and the second being what others are noticing in this person. However, I am an untrained observer and so I use the terms interchangeably.

I show Tony the sections I've written, and he is fine with them in that moment. But of course, he then forgets what he's read.

I can't say for sure this book wasn't my idea. We seemed to reach the decision to write it at the same moment, walking along a beach in February 2017. We discussed it at length during our stay at The Sylvia Hotel, the first pages begun there. Tony thought he had MCI, and while he acknowledged it could worsen, it wasn't until the end of that year that he could agree it had.

Why write this book, then? I suppose we have because Tony was filled with a desire to share our story with the public. When Tony got fired up about the subject, or I did, or later, when he noted the peacefulness that came with a sure diagnosis, we returned to the project with renewed purpose. This is a story worth telling. In those moments when it was most difficult to tell, I was convinced of it. I just wish it wasn't ours.

This is as good a place as any, then, to state that what follows in this book is not meant to ridicule or place blame but to acknowledge what so many of us coping with the dread of Alzheimer's have gone through and, in so doing, provide validation of those experiences. These pages say: Look. Are you seeing the same things in your life or in the life of someone you know? If so, then know that something is wrong. Here's what we did, and maybe you can do it even sooner.

As Tony noted back in 2017:

> Like this journal, my observations will, of course, bounce back and forth in time, in emotion, in observation, and in just about any other way you can imagine. But then of course this is a symptom of the condition, isn't it? (or maybe it's a symptom of how my mind has always worked, and this is simply an attempt to find a description for it.)

At the same time that Tony was experiencing that shift, the start of the "long, slow fade" as he called it, things were changing at home, as well. In 2000 we were still living in our house. Our son had become a high-school graduate and soon moved from the attic to the basement suite, which had its own entrance. We had always encouraged him to move out once he graduated, as our parents had done with us, and he might say now that we were awfully enthusiastic about it. Still, if it wasn't exactly a place of his own, the basement suite at least provided Garth with a gradual immersion into independent living. At one point, he moved out, leaving the two of us rambling about the big old house. We used to say that if I was in the basement and Tony three floors above in the attic, we had to phone each other to meet in the middle for dinner.

That was probably the start of a restlessness in both of us. Tony was always looking for something new, and I was feeling both sad and weary from the role of caregiving for my mother. Part of the reason for my leap from the security of a teaching job to the uncertainty of writing was that I felt I was on borrowed time. What if I inherited Alzheimer's disease? I was in my late forties. Time was running out.

We moved into an apartment in January 2004 after, as I mentioned, we returned from Spain. Downsizing was an economic move, putting more money in the bank to supplement Tony's severance funds and giving me financial freedom to write.

This apartment had high ceilings and large windows, a fireplace, a second bedroom that became Tony's office, a flex space that was my office, and, most important of all, because his green thumb hadn't completely vanished, a rooftop deck where Tony could tend potted plants. Both living and garden spaces were compact, manageable. We made minor adjustments: having the walls painted, the bathroom floor tiled and French doors installed for better air flow. I wanted to wait for another apartment in the building, a north-facing unit, but Tony felt the bright southern exposure of this one would be good for his depression.

We plugged in our computers and got back to work.

Tony landed short-term work in Toronto the following year. We packed up the car with a few possessions, including our dog, and drove across the country. One of Tony's sisters and a niece were in Ontario, and his mother lived out there also. It was good to see more of them. My mother was still in care, but my father managed a trip out to visit us, as did Garth. I used the time there to look for a literary agent and, just before we returned home to Vancouver a couple of months later, I found representation.

When I look back at this two-year period, I am amazed at all the changes, the sheer upheaval. Interestingly, I don't recall this being a bad time for Tony, emotionally or cognitively. The drive to and from Toronto was free of the problems that we experienced in Spain. Was it because we shared the driving this time, our car being an automatic? And work wasn't as much of an issue. Was that because the job was short-term, therefore not as stressful and demanding as a permanent job, allowing that sense of a quick escape? I don't know. It was as though we both needed the adventure. And what he has written about the revitalizing aspects of change, the craving for it, seems to fit that observation.

Once back in Vancouver, things got very busy. I had a novel to finish, and Tony focused on finding more work. Our life seemed to settle down.

An apartment doesn't have the elbow room of a house, though. Tony liked to pace from room to room when he did telephone interviews, and I had nothing but a shoji screen between me and his enthusiastic conversations. If the space was too small for both of us to work comfortably, it was also, perhaps, too quiet. Tony clearly missed the camaraderie of the newsroom, the interaction with others, and all this gave me the idea that he should use some of his earnings to rent office space. It seemed like a good plan, and Tony found a modestly priced office in an old brick building in Vancouver's Gastown district. He loved the space and the opportunity to socialize. He was also getting enough work to keep him busy, and to pay the bills. After about a year, however, the landlord needed the office space and Tony was back to looking for another.

In 2006 my mother died. Tony had been a great support through all the years of care, the agony of putting her into a home, of watching her fade. The following year, I received some money from my mother's estate. It was not a fortune, but given that Tony had received the last of the severance installments, I thought it might put a smile on his face. My novel *Underground* had just been accepted for publication, and he was thrilled for me — so much so I often had to quell his enthusiastic talk at parties when he was about to reveal details of the plot that I wanted kept quiet. But my advance had been small, and I hoped this inheritance would make up for that. It didn't. Tony was even irritated by it.

We talked about this recently. Tony said he was under financial stress.

I said, All the more reason the money should have been welcomed. I added: If a house is going up in flames, do you shout at the person dragging over the hose?

He replied: You do if it's a garden hose.

Touché.

Still, his reaction surprised me. Once more, it seemed out of proportion to the situation. But I was absorbed by many things going on at the same time: revisions for my novel, my father's ill health following a stroke shortly after my mother died, not to mention her death, and I didn't ask Tony what was going on, I mean really going on, to prompt such a response.

During our series of emails, I asked Tony about that period to see if he could recall what he was feeling then.

That time in Toronto, I barely remember it. I can't even remember the name of the guy I worked for and the job.

The big problem for me back then is I didn't know what it was I wanted to do. I was exploring and learning. It was an apprenticeship.

I was entering a major period of depression, too.

I remember the big changes that rocked us in the early 2000s. In fact they were a continuance of the changes that began after we were married and, living a good family life for some time.

But this time I was I my early 50's, probably at the peak of my earning power, and relatively settled in as a husband and stepfather, complete with condo and dog. I had even returned to university, after many years out, and over the nest few years where I was even older than most of my teaches, finished up my degree.

The years of roaming and dreaming wildly and and planning for my future were over. Now I had a real life, and I was going to make the best of it. I worked on the apartment and companion garden as much as I could, and commissioned workmen to do what I couldn't. It turned a relatively plain, not very-well-planned home into an airy condo, that we would now kill for, but at the time, was merely (we thought) a starter place.

I was working. You were working, after some retraining to be a teacher. And we had money. Our condo had appreciated, I was earning and you had begun to earn again after getting a teaching job. We had a lovable , rambunctious dog and a son that was happy — at least most of the time — he was going through the usual teenage angst and depressions.

We had few worries. Except that after a while we both began to get itchy again. You wanted to get back to writing and I wanted a new challenge. Although I had switched jobs, to heading a rewrite desk to becoming a business writer. Where, of course — we first met, and eventually married (which unfortunately led you your being let go — they weren't real keen on couples working together, and found some excuse).

The job was much fun overall. We were a rebellious, crazy, lot who had much fun trying to one-up each other in style, and occasional outrage. We used to give awards to each other every year for the most outrageous, lyrical. hard-boiled, etc.

Sometimes we would pretend it was the1950's and shout "Rewrite" like they used to do in the movies. We sang crazy songs made up by Shane, this genius on the team who loved to write ditties about various characters or events.

Even the editors, some of whom frowned and harrumphed when we first introduced this half hard-news half mad-magazine approach to newspaper writing, got into the act eventually. Although we often crossed the line and shocked some of the older staff, we did sometimes produce amazing gems of short writing. I really believe those were was the best years of my career. Better yet, our antics seemed to vitalize the entire newsroom. Reporters sharpened their writing, Editors tried to outdo each other in producing snappy (and occasionally outrageous) headlines.

But eventually, the conservatives took over and the fun faded. Gradually, it became a production-line job, still busy and occasionally interesting when something big happened, but for the most part, a job where you punched the clock, did your time and got the hell out of there as fast as you could. Like some others, I felt it was as far as I could go and the old restlessness and sadness that had haunted me for most of my life, made a return engagement. The Paper also apparently agreed that it was time for a change and eventually eliminated the entire Rewrite operation, terming it redundant. Of course, it was also a way to downsize staffing — a not uncommon technique in the new world of media.

Figuring that it was coming, I looked for a change to keep myself interested. I moved from reporting to business writing (which, frankly, shocked everybody. But they didn't realize that it was a perfect 9-5 job that would let me have a real life — i.e. family, a little creative writing on the side as well as some freelancing to make some extra money. Also, I started to build a little free-lance writing business.

Meanwhile you were building a teaching career, especially teaching English and writing, which let you feel like you were still on the path to writing. You were also writing more of your own stuff and getting some notice as a writer and a teacher of writing, although that was in its early stages.

It was blissful for a while, but then a recurring desire for a change, or new adventure, in me started to demand attention. You, believe, began again looking for you old love and a desire for a more serious stab at real writing was growing.

31

Here, Tony is "bouncing back and forth," as he told us he would, circling the subject, coming back around to points from the past and then moving forward, then back, and zig-zagging through time as he studies himself and us. There is an impulsivity to this method that is fascinating. He'll have to forgive his linear-thinking wife for trying to connect the dots, and for noting that he skipped over 2006 and 2007 entirely. Really, who says the dots have to be connected and can't simply float? But for the purposes of clarity, I'll mention a few things.

I was dropped by *The Province* in the late 1980s, to my knowledge because I was temporary and had made an error in my copy, and the pressure was always on to either make a temporary worker permanent, or, if the work wasn't ongoing, to end the position. But perhaps the relationship was a further reason. At any rate, it was unnecessary, as I had just handed in my notice. I was leaving work to attend university for my education degree. I wanted to be an English teacher so I could have my summers off to write fiction. This was two homes before we moved to our current apartment.

Tony had been taking courses at university for many years, gradually accumulating enough credits for a Bachelor of Arts degree. I took a photo of his graduation in spring 1994. His niece Alice got her degree on the same day. Garth was about to turn twelve. So, Tony was forty-five years old then.

His employer in 2005 was a man named Ross who lived in Vancouver, but the assignment was in Toronto. Ross was putting together a film series on small businesses in that city that included interviews, with Tony talking, and asking, about various aspects of being an entrepreneur.

During our stay in Toronto, we lived in a small apartment on the ground floor of a brick semi-detached house near Queen Street and Broadview Avenue. The film crew took the cramped space in stride. Bright studio lights lit up the little suite, and there were cables draped all over the furniture and floors. Katie found great pleasure in leaping over everything and barking.

Tony had described Toronto as large and noisy, and my western bias convinced me I wouldn't like it, this place so far from the ocean. We loved it: the red brick, the streetcars, and the fact that a short stroll along Queen Street brought us meat from a butcher and vegetables from a grocer, and even wine from a wine shop, all without the need to step into a busy supermarket. We were surprised that daffodils, which had bloomed in Vancouver in February and March, were only just appearing in May, but the heat of summer arrived quickly by June. We met with family, drove to Ottawa and London to see more family, had dinner with a few of Tony's business associates, and discovered the local passion for tiny blueberries, about half the size of the ones grown out West, but sweeter. As much as I loved the West Coast, I knew I would miss Toronto when we moved back.

Tony did other freelance work while we were there. I never asked what he made in total during our stay there, or what the costs were and how much was covered by the job. Our finances were always an issue, though, even when we didn't talk about it. We drove there and back and stayed in cheap motels because we had our dog with us, and to save money.

We had other money set aside, as I've mentioned. Once my novel was published, I would have the credentials, along with my teaching background, to earn a part-time income teaching writing workshops. In the meantime, Tony had taken out a line of credit to ensure the bills got paid during the ups and downs of freelance work.

It seemed we had everything worked out.

# THE RECESSION'S FAULT, OR IS IT?

On the eve of 2008 a recession loomed. I was particularly aware of the number of businesses in the publishing field that were affected, saw bookstores and small presses close and larger publishing houses amalgamate. Tony worked long hours but never seemed to get ahead. In the past, in addition to working at his office he sometimes spent an evening or weekend at his desk at home, putting a final polish on work, but now the need to do so was constant.

I was always at a loss when asked to explain what exactly Tony did for a living. He set up his own company, Knowpreneur Consultants, and took some courses so that he could work as a consultant for small businesses or entrepreneurial companies, but his role seemed to change with each new contract. Initially, he worked in an advisory role, but frequently he was required to do some writing. He enjoyed a temporary post filling in as the editor for *BC Business*, which was more like his old line of work, and he wrote a regular column for them.

In one piece from early in the year, "Death and Parking: A Stupid Tax Laid to Rest," Tony clearly relished the punchy writing style that was reminiscent of his days in the newsroom. "One of the dumbest concepts ever to come down the pike died a welcome death in the flurry of year-end government cleanups just before Christmas.… This was a classic 'tax-the-rich' concept that could only come out of the woolly-headed thinking of a bunch of small-town dinosaurs caught in some kind of '70s class-war time warp."

Occasionally, Tony also composed in a more serious style, ghostwriting books on business, but the snappy magazine columns provided a steady, modest income.

When Tony freelanced, he would sometimes do a job for free — for the experience, he said, to put something on his resume. Other times, he would begin a job and then tell me that "they" killed the job part way. The reasons were always vague. I would ask if he at least got paid for what he had done, and would then find out that he had not asked for anything up front.

The dark days of winter were drawing in. December 6 is St. Nicholas Day, or what we call Dutch Christmas, and it often stood out from the general gloom as an excuse to throw large house parties. Tony loved them. But Christmas itself, what for others like me was a joyful period of tree-decorating and gift-giving? It had always depressed him. He said his family chose to work during the holidays to earn extra money, so they were not a source of fond memories. This year, however, would turn out to be different.

Vancouver had one of its rare heavy snowfalls, in which the rain-slicked streets became a clogged, frozen, impassable series of narrow pathways. People shovelled to no avail. When a rainforest climate turns cold, there is so much snow. Around our small apartment block alone it took teams of residents digging for several shifts a day to clear the sidewalks.

On December 24, we were supposed to have our traditional get-together with Tony's sister Cinda, her husband, Godwin, and their family. It was also our niece Uche's birthday. Tony strapped chains onto the tires and we drove over to Garth's, where we then drove him and his girlfriend, Joni, and her children to the dinner. It took two shifts to get everyone there because of the number of kids: an older child plus triplets. Tony stopped at a corner piled high with snow to drop off first Leah, Mason, and me. Garth rode back with him for the second run, to help push or shovel if needed.

It was the wrong corner. We didn't realize this until we got out and Tony had already driven away. Was that another sign? Perhaps. Or was it simply that all the snow had made the block unrecognizable? Off we trudged. Our dog Katie turned into fine strutting shape because it seemed that every yard in that South Vancouver neighbourhood, despite the tall drifts of snow, had a pit bull lunging at the fence. I was afraid for the children, but Katie, in true Jack Russell–style, lunged back, determined to protect us all.

By the time we had stomped several blocks in, we were soaked to the knees. We made it there only a few minutes before Tony and Garth, now with Joni and the other two of the triplets, Merrick and Morgan, pulled up, wheels jingling in chains. Tony was smiling broadly: the adventure, the challenge.

I don't know if we had ham that year, a favourite, or the equally delicious beef brisket because family friend Miriam was Jewish and didn't eat ham, but it was the usual crowded, warm, noisy dinner that broke up early only because of the snow. We agreed that we would all stay at our respective homes for Christmas Day itself, as another trip out would be too much.

The next day, Christmas morning, we walked and carried Katie through the snow drifts in our neighbourhood. What gifts did we open? Who knows. We flipped the switch on the gas fireplace and sat by that fire to eat warmed mincemeat tarts with our coffee. We watched old Christmas movies on TV, as well as the classic *Casablanca*, with Humphrey Bogart — also Dutch, Tony reminded me — and Ingrid Bergman.

During commercials, I leapt up to stir the gravy and heat the cranberry sauce. I set the table with our best china plates and silverplated flatware, our crystal wine glasses and linen napkins, and lit the candles. It was a modest dinner by Christmas standards, just roasted turkey breast served with minimal sides, like mashed potatoes, stuffing, and salad. We had Christmas carols playing in the background. Our old dog consumed her fair share of turkey, too. After, we walked Katie again, just around the building as it was very cold and she was shivering, then we raced back in to the fire and the warmth and watched more movies. Much like that two-year time of upheaval, I don't recall this snowfall and the arduous four trips, driving back and forth, to be a bad time for Tony, emotionally or cognitively. Had we not seen everyone the night before, we would have missed the presence of family, but as it was, it was such a simple, quiet Christmas — full of warmth and food and drink and our dog curled up with us and Humphrey Bogart — that it remains a favourite for both of us. Most important of all, and this is something I am only now realizing, it had provided Tony with a badly needed break from what was becoming a nightmare of a working life. I knew he was struggling, but I did not fully realize that it was taking its toll on his cognitive well-being. Not yet, at least.

In the new year, things went back to where they had been before December. Tony began to talk increasingly of jobs he had started that were suddenly pulled — more fallout from the recession that spilled over into 2009. We were both upset that once again people didn't pay him for the half that had been done. I also grew concerned that more than one accused him of being sloppy. First drafts always are, and we talked about people's ignorance of the collaborative spirit of writing — that it's a process that thrives on feedback and editing and so on. Still, I wondered, should he have been showing drafts as rough as that?

I didn't pursue it. I was preoccupied. My father was needing more help, and the family emergencies and late-night calls were exhausting. Garth's paternal grandfather had just died. Bob was not only family but a good friend, and the loss hit us hard. I was also juggling my own writing career and revisions for *Underground.* The novel was published in March, and I grew busy with ensuing readings and teaching jobs. Tony and I were absorbed in our own worlds, trying to make inroads in our careers, trying to earn enough money to pay the bills. Where we found agreement was over concern for our old and now ailing dog Katie.

She died mid-year, and Tony and I decided the best thing to do was to walk out our grief. We walked everywhere: neighbourhood walks, half-day walks, under the blistering sun of summer, into the rainy fall; we walked without a leash in our hands, without the need to rush home to feed her or let her out. Eventually, by the end of the year, we grew accustomed to life without her. Some of you will be nodding with understanding as you read this. Pets are part of the family. Others may wonder how the loss of the family dog can have greater impact than the loss of loved ones. But Tony has said many times that she was an integral part of our early years with our son, so her death marked a final end of that life and a true beginning of the aging process in ourselves.

Six months later, at the start of 2010, I received grant money and spent the next six months working on my second novel.

During this time, Tony hired both a business coach and an office manager, who would work remotely, to help him find work and keep a schedule. I hadn't thought about how difficult it must have been for a former news reporter, so used to being assigned stories, to have to drum up ideas himself and keep organized. I asked him if he, with only his regular business column to count on, could afford the expense of hiring anyone? He replied that he was following the advice that you have to spend money to make money.

Tony's mother had been diagnosed with cancer a few years earlier, and in the fall, she died. I thought the slump in Tony, the lack of spark, was grief. There had been so many losses in a row. Also, she had taken her own life rather than endure the pain of a long, slow death, and while we admired her courage, it also shook us, or perhaps it shook me. Tony says the Dutch are more practical than the sentimental English.

As I had, following the death of my mother, Tony received a small inheritance, and since we hadn't travelled out of the country for seven years and were suddenly free of the task of finding someone to dog-sit, I suggested a two-week trip after Christmas. Again, family and work came together. Tony's niece Alice had invited us to visit her in Hong Kong, where we could stay for free in her friend's apartment, and I could do research for my second novel, stopping in Shanghai on the way home, where we were scheduled to transfer planes anyway.

What an adventure it was. Hong Kong: so much like Vancouver, and yet not — more San Francisco–like, with its steep streets and narrow, twisting alleys; like nothing else in its lush scenery, its crowds, its food. Tony was impressed with Mong Kok, one of the most densely populated places on earth, but on New Year's Eve, a chance to ring in 2011 in Hong Kong, he wanted to go back to the apartment and stay in. From the confines of our flat, we watched digitally projected fireworks race up the sides of the high-rises around us, heard the vague, distant roar of cheers from the streets below.

Tony livened up in Shanghai, where we rode in a motorcycle and sidecar, as research, we said, but it was pure fun. Tony used to ride a motorcycle, and it must have brought back memories. We drank cocktails at the Glamour Bar on the Bund and took a bullet train to Suzhou, where I gave a reading at the Suzhou Bookworm. This event had been arranged through a connection of the Vancouver Writers Festival. I had appeared at the festival the year before, and when artistic director Hal Wake heard where I was heading for research, he got in touch with a friend. The Worm staff were wonderful hosts, feeding us and providing accommodation in a nearby hotel. The chef, Ben, took time out of his schedule to walk us around Suzhou, a city of pretty canals and ancient dwellings.

During the vacation, Tony came down with a cold, but before we caught our flight home I tried to coax him out one last time. Again, he wanted to stay in. But we were in Shanghai! Our last night! We had to eat something, so we went to a local cafe serving bland food. We ate half-heartedly until Justin Bieber appeared on the gigantic electronic wall screen, singing "Baby, baby, baby, oh," and the two young servers raced over to dance below the image, bursting into song, too.

We kept pointing to the screen and then to ourselves, saying, Same. Canadian. I'm sure the young women wondered what on earth the two old geezers were trying to say about themselves and the cute Bieber, and ignored us. We walked home that last night laughing and, okay, who could resist, singing that chorus. It is a moment I cherish because things were about to change dramatically.

When I told Tony what section I was working on, and that it went back ten years, he asked to see it. This was in early 2018. The process we were using involved me piecing together the narrative based on our 2017 emails. I would write, and he would respond. This time was different, as the following response shows. He wasn't present in that snowy scene with our dog lunging at the pit bulls — he had already driven off in the car — yet he has put himself into the scene.

I am leaving it in as an example of a mis-memory that is consistent with the disease, and is perhaps also reflective of his desire to share that memory. This sort of borrowing is there, too, in the opening lines of this email: His quotation of lyrics from a Maurice Chevalier song is influenced by another 2018 email exchange between Tony and me that I will be quoting in full later in the book. Eventually, I would make the decision to no longer show him pieces in progress. Instead, I would have him write his thoughts separately, first, then I would weave them into the text, giving him the final result to read. This is another example of my concerns about my role in this project. In this instance, I am not just directing the story's progress but shifting the course of one narrative thread. I have to believe such a correction is what Tony would want. In the passage below, when he moves into a description of the assignments that were going wrong, he fully owns the memory and the associated feelings. They spring from his recollection, alone, and reinforce my decision that this is how all of his entries should be, written independently of mine with their potential to unduly influence.

Hmm … 2008 … I remember that turn of the year — (I believe that I'm starting to sound like that guy in the Maurice Chevalier song duet "I Remember It Well" when she corrected him on some long-ago event.)

At least I do now, that I read your notes. I couldn't remember the details until I read it — and I'm amazed that you remembered it all.

However ... As I (cough, cough) ... recall, that was the recession when my work, and, apparently, my mind, started to founder.

But then, as always seems to be the case ... it was also in some ways a great year.

Our little dog Katie was true to form, snarling protection when the pitbull next door to my sister's place made some noise — as he should have since he was supposed to be a watchdog, which was needed in that neighbourhood.

But Katie was a cocky little thing, a true Jack Russel Terrier ("come on, I can take him just let me at him!") and lunged back at him when he made a move. At least we managed to pry her away from the fence before he tore her up (which other victims of her "safekeeping" actions had come closer to doing).

It was a wild day, more like some day way up north than down here in Lotus Land. Snow up to our knees, and most people around us not knowing what to do, and certainly not knowing how to drive in the snow!

But inside, it was all warmth and *Gemutlichkeit* with our usual Jewish/Catholic/Protestant/ Christmas crew at my sister's. The African, Dutch, Jewish Christmas was a hit. Thank god for the tire chains, which, for some reason, only my vague memories of snowstorms experienced when I was a kid prompted me to bring them along.

Try that now! I'd be lucky to remember to wear boots.

Anyway, it was easily one of the best Christmases I have ever been lucky to be part of. Those kind of post-card events — watching Casablanca and singing the French anthem with the french people in the pictured pub that had been invaded by Nazi soldiers — stay with you forever.

Unfortunately, that was the high point. Other events of the time were not so nice. I was clearly having problems with my work, which, I presume in retrospect, were the result of encroaching "brain farts" as we in the newsroom called memory gaps.

But I didn't see them as that at the time. My writing business, which I had launched with great hopes and an avalanche of work, wasn't living up to expectations. Okay, it was foundering like a leaky canoe.

I couldn't understand why I was getting complaints from clients that I was sloppy, or hadn't included something, or was off track. I partly attributed it to the fact that many of the clients didn't understand the process — that writing a book was an ongoing thing, and didn't just spring perfectly on to the page after an outline that wasn't even a first draft.

We were dealing with some complicated stuff here (usually advisory books on business operation by consultants who wanted to use them for marketing purposes) which takes some time and much discussion. But they didn't seem to understand that I couldn't just do some basic research and whip up a hundred pages or so, without much input from them.

I tried to explain this, and in a few cases that worked. But too often it didn't, or I didn't explain it well. They had agreed to the process, and expected that the process would just appear. One soon — to be ex-client even complained that I had conned her. "I thought I was hiring this great writer," she shouted at me, "and instead I got THIS!" That really hurt.

Some did managed to stagger to success, but others foundered or didn't even start. Soon, I was continually focusing on the problems and complaints instead of the rare successes. This ghost writing career was not exactly going as expected — a mini business correction at the time didn't help either — and I was essentially existing on free-lance journalism and borrowing to pay the bills.

My confidence was sinking, and I was becoming more unfocused and tired, which I attributed to tension and the usual business ups and downs in order to keep going. Also, I was learning a new business, one where I was often put in the place of the servant , the hireling, and not the inquisitor or interviewer, a familiar place for me. Maybe it was just a case of better adapting to the landscape. Or ameliorating my personality to better fit the new role. Or maybe we were just speaking different languages that added to the misalignment of purposes.

My ego and confidence — my swagger — continued to shrink. For perhaps a year or more, I oscillated between anger and despair, with despair winning. I couldn't understand what was happening, and worse, I couldn't find any way to reverse it. Previously, I had been able to analyze and change my thinking if it was preventing what I wanted to do.

When I did pull off some good stuff, usually my columns or my business writing, it was like strapping on a well-worn, comfortable harness that had fitted my body and mind over time. But when I stepped out of harness, I was confused, lost, angry ... and afraid.

People — potential clients, others connected with the business, etc. — began to avoid me. I' went to fewer and fewer industry events where I should have been marketing my services, but instead found myself sitting in corners or sending all my time with only a few people and secretly lamenting the fact that I was a terrible businessman. People didn't feel the need to talk with me any more — in my mind, because I couldn't do anything for them, and, generally, in the business world, if you aren't useful, you don't exist.

Somehow I had become tainted. But I couldn't understand why or how. What had I done wrong?

That client had been horrible to Tony. Even so, given the other jobs that had fizzled, I did wonder what might have happened in the writing of the project to prompt such a rude outburst, and if it was the result of her misunderstanding, or his. It is also interesting to note that, despite the memory gaps that include not even mentioning his mother's death, Tony has not forgotten the sting of that client's rebuke.

# PART TWO

---

# THE JOURNEY BEGINS

# THE FALL

Late January in 2011 must have been snowless, the complete opposite of that winter two years before when we had to strap chains onto the tires to drive a mere few blocks within East Vancouver.

We had just returned from China, and after a few days of re-adjusting to our familiar time zone, I headed out for dinner with Terri, who was living in Vancouver again. On such evenings, Tony often visited next door with our neighbour Richard, or sat by the fire watching a movie.

If every moment I have described until now has been a shift, a slight change, a ripple on the surface of our normal lives, the one this evening was cataclysmic.

I came home around midnight. The fire was roaring in the gas fireplace and a bottle of brandy stood open on the counter. I head-ed up onto the roof, thinking Tony was upstairs having a cigar. The roof was empty, though, so I returned, a little concerned that he had gone off to Richard's and left the fireplace on. Then I saw the flashing light on our home phone and snatched it up. It was a message from Tony saying that he'd had a fall in the kitchen and had taken a cab to Emergency. I called him back and got his voice mail. I raced around the counter of the open kitchen and only then saw a large pool of blood on the floor. I have no recollection of cleaning the floor, though I must have at some point, or of turning off the fireplace. I grabbed the car keys and headed outside.

That's how I know it wasn't snowing. We no longer drive when it snows, as we've never bothered with the expense of snow tires, and the chains were too much trouble.

Burnaby Hospital is within walking distance, but I was in a hurry, and it was late.

Tony wasn't there.

I tried his phone again. Nothing. I wondered if he had gone to Vancouver General Hospital, instead, or St. Paul's, or Mount Saint Joseph Hospital. I had just got back in the door when the home phone rang, and it was Tony, on his way back from VGH with a few stitches in his chin.

At first, I thought he'd had too much to drink. So did he, and I'm sure I said something critical about that. Only there wasn't that much brandy gone from the bottle. Over the next couple of days I began questioning him. I thought he might have had a stroke. How much had he had to drink? Was there wine as well? He couldn't recall. Did they give him an X-ray at Emergency? A CT scan? Again, he couldn't recall.

Over the next few weeks and months, I noticed he was leaving stove elements on.

This sort of thing had happened before, and back then I wasn't overly alarmed. One time, he butted out a cigar in one of the potted plants on our deck, heedless of the fact that it was full of peat moss, and that he'd started a mini bog-fire. I'd only discovered it because my office was right below the opened skylight, and it had filled with smoke. I was annoyed with him for not knowing better. He was a gardener, after all.

My office, as I've mentioned, is divided from the kitchen by a shoji screen, and one time when I was at my desk I heard an odd crackling sound, then saw a brightness through the screen. I leapt up and ran into the kitchen. Tony was sitting at the breakfast bar, reading, oblivious to the flames that crackled from inside a greased pot he had set on the stove and forgotten about. I yelled. Tony ran to the sink, planning to throw water onto the flames. No! I said. The flames could jump the pot and start a kitchen fire. I pushed past him, slammed the lid onto the pot to snuff out the flames, then ran up the stairs to the roof garden where I planted the hot pot into the deep snow to cool it.

So, the latter incident must have been back during that snowy winter of 2008/2009. But although it occurred before my suspicions about Tony's mental state became more serious, the incident troubled me. It seemed amazing that he had forgotten about the dangers of throwing water onto an oil fire. As noted, though, post-2011 and his fall, leaving stove elements on became a regular occurrence, not a rare one.

I insisted he see his doctor. That fall in the kitchen, I said. Maybe you had a stroke. He insisted on going alone and returned saying the doctor had checked him over and he was fine.

And it seemed that he was. By summer, he was writing a regular column for the *Financial Post*, another for *BC Business*, and a season of blogs for CBC's *The Dragon's Den*.

And yet.

Over the next year, he burned through another pot; as well, he closed the barbecue and covered it without turning the elements off, melting the cover until it sealed the unit inside. Tony was at work when I discovered this. He had grilled a chicken lunch to take with him.

I was officially alarmed now.

I would have been even more alarmed had I known that he had stopped filing his GST. However, I didn't know this at the time.

We have discussed his fall and the ensuing events many times. I knew he would not be unduly influenced by my words as it was not new ground for him and so, one last time, I agreed to him reading my words before writing his own. It is difficult for any of us to remember an event from seven years back, but the intermittency of cognitive function in his reply is notable, that he can struggle to recall and to write coherently one minute, then use words plucked from an impressive vocabulary in the next. It's like an electrical wire shorting out, then reconnecting, and it reminds me of what I have had to remind others: having Alzheimer's doesn't make a person stupid. Tony still had and has the knowledge he once had, the vocabulary, too; it's just that his brain can be unpredictable; he is no longer able to rely on it to release the information.

And of course, his reply contains the repetitions that are indicative of the disease.

> Well, that's quite a litany of change. Falls, injuries, black-outs, heavy drinking (which I still believe led to the fall, although I am sure it had some impact on the overall situation). I confess, when I see this, I think (as best as possible now) of how obstreperous I was at the time. Obviously, I was worried too, or I wouldn't have been so secretive.
>
> Instead, I think I was confused at the time. Nothing seemed to be working. My once prolific (I thought) abilities were obviously fading, and it wasn't because I was so much older — I wasn't.

I was seriously depressed because my business was failing, and several people had complained about my work. Frankly, I was acting weird — and, often, angry and it was being commented on, not only by you, but by others. The comments were becoming every faster and ever louder.

In a nutshell (an appropriate word I thought at the time), I was a becoming a mental — and physical wreck, and I couldn't find anybody to blame for it except for myself, which made me even more depressed. What happened to the once-vibrant (at least in my view) man I one was? Where did all my vaunted smarts and stick-to-it determination go? It seem much more drastic than a midlife crisis — I had already bought and then sold the sports car long ago. I had no dreams at all. No plans, no directions, no hopes.

Also, it wasn't like I was 75 and having an end-of-life pondering crisis. (looking back, I should have had one. It would have had a wonderful effect on me. As the Stoics said, Momento Mori - always remember that you will die and it could at any moment).

Only in my 50's, I felt I had no dreams, no plans, no directions, no hopes. I had lost my sense of self. I believe I was self-aware enough to realize this might be more than a severe case of of midlife-change blues that would eventually fade away away as I found my place in this new grown-up-guy world. — but I stuck with that because I couldn't believe that it could be anything else, and certainly not something to do with my brain, which had always been my best and most helpful companion, if not always my best friend (i.e, depression).

Anyway, enough of the memory-lane brooding. You list a series of events that had you worried. — leaving stoves on, starting little fires, and of course, the big one — falling on my face, cutting my chin open and having to grab a cab to what I thought was the nearest hospital (which, for some reason, I had enough brains left to remember — nothing like a crisis to focus the mind. But in my addled state, I got that wrong, But, hey, I did leave you a partial message — which, of course, made things even worse.)

But, as we both now know, that was the beginning of the unexpected downward slide. I was leaving stove elements on, as you observed — worriedly. I was angry more often. I was brooding. the mistakes became more common — and more dangerous, as in leaving the barbecue on, brooding constantly — misremembering, worrying and angry, and sometimes, just not making sense, as in the repetitive behaviours and looping. I definitely couldn't work or write anything. I just mostly read and walked around.

Even in my stupidity, I had some sense of understanding and knew that clearly something was wrong. But I didn't have a clue as to what it was. And I was certain that I couldn't possibly have a brain problem. I thought it was some lingering concussion, like football players get (yeah, that's it, something heroic like that, I tried to convince myself —but failed.)

Even I knew that something was wrong, but I didn't have a clue as to what it was. To say it was just a major depression was clearly understating it. Although I tried not to show it, and may even have succeeded some of the time, I was really, really worried.

Again, I sent him to his doctor and, again, he insisted on going alone. He must have described either my concern or the burning pots, or both, because this time the doctor referred him to a specialist, a gerontologist. But it can take months to see a specialist, and the appointment would not take place until the following year.

It was 2012. Tony was back to working from home now, to conserve funds and also because he complained to me that he kept falling asleep at his desk, which alarmed me. His younger sister had just had a stroke, and, once more, I wondered if he had had one, too. They were so much alike, it seemed possible, except that Cinda had been left with such typical aftereffects as impaired speech. She also found it difficult to retrieve words, even if she knew what she wanted to say. For instance, she might try to say the word *brother*, but, instead, she'd say *son*, then she'd try to correct herself by saying their names, and flop those as well. Tony, on the other hand, was as loquacious as ever.

My mother, years before her diagnosis of Alzheimer's disease, had had a fall, too. A later brain scan would reveal signs of ministrokes. But I still chose to not connect those dots. I chose to focus instead on the possibility that Tony had had a stroke.

Garth and Joni married on December 23, a magical evening with streets decorated in Christmas lights and many of us in cocktail attire. The bride wore a white gown straight out of a storybook and was walked down the aisle by her four children. We became instant grandparents, though we had unofficially enjoyed that role for years.

We took in two of Garth and Joni's cats: a ginger kitten the previous summer and then, several months after the wedding, a grey tabby, both strays that had shown up at their doorstep when they already had two cats. Tony loved animals, and it never occurred to any of us that the presence of pets could be a challenge.

One night, after the cats' arrival, I was out with our friend Terri. I returned to find a row of dishes of water lined up along the wall, which was an unusual sight. I wish I had recorded the date, because for all I know this happened the following year. Is this important? Yes and no. Yes, because I am trying to track the early signs, and would like to get them in the right order. I hadn't started writing things down yet. If it was 2013, then Tony was under sixty-five years of age, the cut-off for young-onset Alzheimer's disease, an issue I will discuss further at the end of the book. And no, because it had to be within a year or so of getting the cats, as Tony soon left their care up to me, and that's close enough.

On this night, instead of feeding the cats, Tony had picked up their dishes, headed into the kitchen, and filled them with water. When he put the dishes down, he must have known something was wrong, because there was already a water fountain for them, but he went and got more dishes, this time saucers, then filled them with water, too; and then again. It wasn't that he had forgotten to feed the cats, exactly, but halfway through the process of picking up their dishes, something in his brain switched off, and when he tried again, it switched off again, and then again. It was as though the minute he touched the objects, their purpose vanished, or they shape-shifted into something else, turning from food dishes into water dishes. Again, I imagined an electrical wire shorting out, only in this case even the presence of several vessels of water triggered no corrective thoughts, no reconnecting of that wire.

I came home to two very hungry cats and a perplexed Tony, who stared at the row of dishes of water as though seeing them for the first time.

It was around then that, with much trepidation, I began looking up those lists: "Ten Warning Signs of Alzheimer's Disease." Here is one from the Alzheimer Society of Canada:

1.  **Memory loss affecting day-to-day abilities** — forgetting things often or struggling to retain new information.
2.  **Difficulty performing familiar tasks** — forgetting how to do something you've been doing your whole life, such as preparing a meal or getting dressed.
3.  **Problems with language** — forgetting words or substituting words that don't fit the context.
4.  **Disorientation in time and space** — not knowing what day of the week it is or getting lost in a familiar place.
5.  **Impaired judgment** — not recognizing a medical problem that needs attention or wearing light clothing on a cold day.
6.  **Problems with abstract thinking** — not understanding what numbers signify on a calculator, for example, or how they're used.
7.  **Misplacing things** — putting things in strange places, like an iron in the freezer or a wristwatch in the sugar bowl.
8.  **Changes in mood and behaviour** — exhibiting severe mood swings from being easy-going to quick-tempered.
9.  **Changes in personality** — behaving out of character such as feeling paranoid or threatened.
10. **Loss of initiative** — losing interest in friends, family and favourite activities.[*]

Was this issue a sign of #2? Or #5? Or #7? Not exactly. I had been hoping to be proved wrong, and this list seemed to do that. Tony's behaviour didn't quite fit any of these, though #8, changes in mood and behaviour, had me thinking of Pamplona. I honestly don't know why #10, loss of interest, didn't remind me of the garden or the newsroom. I suppose I was focused on what the

---

[*] This and all subsequent quotes from Alzheimer Society Canada are copyrighted as indicated here: © March 2020. Alzheimer Society of Canada. All rights reserved. alzheimer.ca.

row of dishes meant. The familiar task (#2) was partly performed. Judgment (#5) was impaired in that the contents got mixed up, but the dishes themselves remained clearly cats' dishes that belonged on the floor, so he hadn't misplaced them (#7), and even saucers are typically used as cat dishes, and were in a neat row. What bothered me was that he couldn't see the problem as it lay there in front of him, dish after dish of water, and the cats turning figure eights about his ankles, crying for food. What did that mean?

No, I thought, almost hopefully, he must have had a stroke of some sort, different from his sister's. That would explain the shorting out, what I was beginning to see as "dead time" in the middle of otherwise normal moments. I wanted desperately for it to be a stroke, because improvement through rehabilitation was then possible. As I knew from my mother's illness, there is no recovery from Alzheimer's.

But really, who was I kidding? I knew the signs.


Tony's first appointment with the gerontologist, I should add, was in the spring of 2013. I have no details of it to record here because, once more, Tony insisted on going on his own. It was the same for a psychiatrist he had been seeing over a number of years for depression.

Why didn't I go with him anyway? My father was in his eighties, with vascular dementia, and our calendar was crammed with appointments for him, for medical, financial, housing, and other concerns, as they had been for years since my mother's death. In the month of March alone, there were six of them. My brother helped for a while but his health was failing — he would end up needing heart surgery. Eventually, I would hire a driving service to give me some relief. Even then, I was swamped. So, I thought, if Tony didn't want me along for his appointments, fine, I would let it go. At the time, he felt that he was fine, and again, certainly there were times he seemed just fine.

As he noted in 2017, he had always been somewhat disorganized and creative, so in that respect the husband I was seeing four years earlier was the same old Tony.

> Let's face it — I'm a putter-together of thoughts, not a planner of thoughts — for very long, my mind has been an endless stream of thoughts, with one after another popping up and sending me off on a trail of other thoughts related to the subject — like a dog following a scent (and, then looking up and discovering he is lost in the woods, etc. ).
>
> I was always this way — a dreamer they called me, always thinking of something airy-fairy, of what could be done instead of what had to be done, always exploring, and , unfortunately, always exploring myself. This usually resulted in sadness — of my background, of my inabilities, of my future, of opportunities lost, of opportunities that won't happen, of blocks to my desires and dreams and explorations. In short I was a dreamer and a depressive. As far back as I can remember.

The gerontologist, bless her, was firm about Tony bringing me along next time. Unfortunately, next time would be a full year later, in 2014.

# PANIC

In early 2014, we received notice of unpaid bills — five months of them. This meant that back in the fall of 2013, Tony had simply stopped making payments.

Tony had always taken care of the finances because his world was financial writing and he could run some of the household bills through his business. I had been busy dealing with my father and his affairs (I shared power of attorney (POA) with my sister, Pam, but she lived out of town). And yet, here we were, behind on payments in every single area possible in our own finances. I was struck by the irony. I was also sickened by it.

I asked Tony what was going on, and he said it was because we didn't have enough money to pay the bills. This made no sense. Pay some of them, if there isn't enough for all bills. But to pay none of them, and for month after month, racking up a debt? This just wasn't like him.

A sense of panic filled me.

Money. I can pretend it's not important, but that would be a lie. True, we all know that money can't buy happiness. There are examples everywhere. But a lack of it can bring misery. You can't pay bills with nothing. You can't buy food with nothing. We don't need a lot of money, but we do need some. From my reckoning, we at least had some, but if we didn't act quickly, the debt would consume it and we would end up with nothing.

I said I would take over the household finances, and Tony was fine with that, saying he found them annoying anyway. I had left the room before I considered what an unusual response this was for him, who had found numbers, especially those attached to dollars, endlessly fascinating. Then again, it was not unusual for him to be depressed about money, and in that context his response made sense.

According to Tony, the psychiatrist had noted as much about the source of his depression and anxiety, and had put him on escitalopram for anxiety and buproprion for depression. I still had not met his psychiatrist, except over the phone when he called to say that Tony hadn't shown up for an appointment. That had seemed a good opportunity for a quick chat, but he had no time and was only interested in getting Tony over there before his office closed.

As for Tony's reaction to the unpaid bills, back then I didn't have time to ponder it any further. I had a lot of work ahead of me to clear up this debt. I would do it, little by little, but it would be more than a year before I would be able to pay everything off.

It was only after we began *Four Umbrellas* that I asked Tony for his thoughts on the whole issue of forgotten bills. In one of his emails, he wrote:

> I am becoming, as my mother used to stay when they gave her too many pills, "STUPID."

I don't remember things. I forget what I was saying half way through a sentence, or I forget a word I was going to use, so have to cover myself by using something else – which may or may not be what I was originally thinking. Now, I do cover this occasionally, and, I suspect, not very convincingly. But it is …. Vexing (a great word).

Don't even ask me about people's names. I don't know anyone's name any more. Heck, I barely remember my own! Just a joke.. I remember my name it's Antonius something or other. Suffice to say this is a problem and I have to do some fancy dancing when I meet someone I know, because I often haven't a clue what their name is. So I plunge in with a "Hi, how are you doing", and then, , bringing up things that I think might give me a trigger – i.e., I often know how I know them, so talk a bit about common interests, hoping that their name will be revealed. Sometimes I carry on entire conversations, and they never realize I can't remember who the are. Other times I devise some ruse, ie need to make a note to someone else, so that they have to give me their name. This can backfire badly, of course.

Other times, if it's someone I haven't seen for a while, I'll just look puzzled, and they'll jump in with their name. This only works with some people- ie people I have interviewed, only met once or twice, or are friends of friends.

April arrived, and this time I went with him to see the gerontologist.

When she asked if I had noted any differences in Tony, she got an earful. I told her everything I could think of. It was a long list: burning elements and barbecues and unpaid bills. The cat dishes!

She seemed almost amused. I stressed that this was Tony we were talking about. Tony was a financial writer. This was five months of forgetting, which was highly unusual for him. If I wasn't shouting then, I'm shouting in my head, now, as I write this.

Another doctor was there, under her mentorship, and they gave Tony the MoCA, the usual memory test, and it showed some cognitive gaps, but, they said, nothing to be too concerned about. For many people, this was a normal score.

The tests were new to me then, and I didn't think to ask what the score was. I now know that it must have been twenty-six out of thirty or higher if they saw no serious concerns. But even from where I was sitting, I could see that his attempt at drawing a three-dimensional cube looked more like a squashed church steeple, and while I didn't yet realize what such visual errors could mean, I knew it wasn't normal. Later, I would test myself to be certain. For now, I was disappointed. I was angry. *I* was depressed. What about all the examples I'd given them? Did those count for nothing?

They were enough, at least, to warrant a follow-up visit.

The gerontologist's next remark, however, was the most frightening thing I could imagine. She turned to me and said, See you in a year.

I fought back tears. I felt as though my head would explode. She acknowledges now that we were in crisis. But back then, she was looking at a patient who presented well and scored within the normal range. Even as they were chatting, Tony waxed eloquent on the state of American politics.

A year!

And what a year it was.


A month after this appointment my father died, following a brief battle with cancer and a longer one with vascular dementia. My sister flew down, and together we settled his affairs. With that experience in mind, I suggested to Tony that we have the lawyer draw up a POA document for both of us. While our recent financial upsets were at the top of my mind, I had to admit that I was thinking that having one parent with Alzheimer's and the other with dementia meant I stood an equally good chance of becoming financially incompetent and would need Tony as my POA.

That gave me pause. I had the lawyer add our son as backup.

The process would not be completed until October, when we would sign for each other and I would file the papers away for future use. I knew from my parents' situations that many banks require a letter from a doctor to activate the POA. We still did not have a diagnosis for Tony. Even so, I felt better with those documents in place.

In the meantime, the memory problems became more than forgotten dates and bills. One night, I awoke at 2 a.m. with a startling thought: Had Tony turned the barbecue off? That was always his responsibility, yet, as I lay there, I couldn't stop thinking about the melted barbecue cover. I got out of bed and crept up the stairs in my nightie, shivering, and rounded the corner to see orange tongues against the black sky. Instead of turning it off, he had turned it up, and left the lid wide open. All it would have taken was a piece of paper fluttering by in the breeze, catching the tip of the flame and then falling onto the wooden deck ... I turned off the elements and the tank and then closed the lid and crept back downstairs.

And there were other things.

My friend Mary Beth began to make jokes. That Tony! she'd say when she called me. Didn't he give you my message? I called twice before.

Richard made similar comments. He has the worst memory! he'd say.

Tony was losing the ability to remember, certainly, but he was also losing the ability to organize, to record important dates, or to check his agenda for dates he'd actually recorded. He was not able to comment in any detail on many past events because he couldn't recall them, but he could write about his condition in the present.

> There is certainly no denying that my mind is not as sharp as it once was. But, on the other hand it is more "dreamy" and "thoughtful" which, from an artistic point of view, is wonderful. It is very much like when I was young and was constantly "lost in thought" or, as my mother said, had "my head in the clouds." I was constantly pestering her with the craziest questions about odd things — what is life?, Do angels get older", how does electricity work, etc. (although I now think they probably weren't as crazy as indicated). She would get so frustrated and angry with me. But I was then able to go back and do deep math or science or reading. (probably because it was all around me, i.e. in school, with my older sister, etc. and because the puzzle and adventure of it all fascinated me.)

It was our twenty-fifth anniversary that August in 2014. I gave Tony a vintage silver coin since silver is the traditional gift for the twenty-fifth. It was also intended as a teasing nod to his love of money. I wasn't expecting a gift in return. We had never made a big fuss of anniversaries, and the coin was small, as gifts go, but I thought he might offer some sort of recognition of the milestone. A card, dinner out, perhaps.

He said, Why bother, it isn't much of a marriage anyway.

I was crushed.

I know now that he was trying to cover for the fact that he had forgotten, and not just forgotten the anniversary date, but the significance of it. He was embarrassed, and in his rush to cover for the mistake he made a worse one without realizing it. And why didn't I see that? I had been noting the repetitions, the forgetfulness.

Well, because emotions overpower logic. The remark stung, even though I knew it shouldn't. He was my closest friend, and the comment was a betrayal of that friendship.

Cinda and Godwin wouldn't hear of us not celebrating, and took us out for dinner, not knowing what had just gone on. It was a beautiful and yet awful dinner, at the former Beach House, now the Fish House, where we had been married.

The following weekend, my niece Kathryn, who is my sister's daughter and has her dark hair and green eyes, was getting married, so for the time being I pushed away Tony's remark. We flew to Prince George for the ceremony, while Garth and his gang drove up. We all stayed in the hotel and had a wonderful time. We went out to see their horses, as well as their cats and dogs. It was good of them to take the time, given how busy they were with wedding arrangements, and with Ron's mom, who was not well and had to be taken to the hospital.

Ron's birthday was coming up and we had brought him a card. I did the usual, filled out the card and signed my name leaving room for Tony to add a few words and his name. Instead, he signed it *June* right under where I had signed, so that it was now inscribed from *June* and *June*.

I held the card in my hands, thinking about that list of ten warning signs. This wasn't on there, either. It did, however, put his comment from the week before into perspective, and I asked him about it. He was surprised, and did not recall saying anything about our marriage. My thoughts were pulled in two directions. This, signing with my name, was a glaring error, and it shook me. It also required correcting, but we had no time before our flight. I got him to simply cross out one *June* and write *Tony* under it. We gave Ron the card, but I've often wondered since if they noticed the mistake. I asked Pam recently and, I suppose in all the wedding details, she hadn't. I certainly hadn't drawn her attention to it. She was the mother of the bride and this wasn't the time to mention my growing suspicions about Tony.

In fact, at this point, Cinda and Garth were the only ones I had discussed Tony's condition with, and Garth and Joni were the only ones who expressed concerns about problems in his memory.

A few weeks later, Tony made a fuss of my September birthday. I suppose the guilt of both forgetting the anniversary and then lashing out to cover it up must have nested itself into his head because several times the following April he burst into the room, in a clear panic about possibly having forgotten, asking, Is it your birthday?

It was a sweet forgetfulness that hurt more than the lashing out. He must have drawn a parallel to April, a month that is a given name, as is my name, *June*.

In early 2015, we flew to Toronto for the traditional Nigerian naming ceremony of our niece Chi-Chi and her husband Kareem's baby boy. Except for Tony's repeated questions about when we would land and what day he was supposed to see his editor at the *Post*, the flight went well. Tony took part in the naming ceremony with Godwin without missing a beat. He had neglected to write a speech, but, as I've mentioned, he is a talker and was able to wing it.

I was seeing an acquaintance the day Tony had to meet his editor. It was bitterly cold, about minus thirty-three degrees Celsius, and I offered to go with Tony, first. But he refused. He had a map and showed me the route he would take. Anthony and I were touring the printing operations at Coach House Press as research for my second novel, and then we went for lunch. It was all within a short distance of the hotel, so I was home before Tony. The wait seemed long, but for all my worrying he made it back on his own. That is the sporadic nature of the failing brain: despite his forgetfulness and repetition of questions on the plane, he could navigate the streets of an unfamiliar city. But then, he knew Toronto from his young adulthood, so he was using old memory. With cognitive decline, old memory can be razor-sharp; in fact, the older, the sharper. It's yesterday's that's dull.

# SAY IT AGAIN, AND AGAIN

I get wild, a lttle crazy, sometimes argumentative, etc. when things don't seem to work, or when things are thrown at me that I can't figure out. This, I think, may account for a lot of our recent set-to's. I'm not sure why, but I'm guessing these moments of panic are one reason – am "oh no, I forgot – again"; or why are you attacking me for something I supposedly did or didn't do, when I don't know what you're talking about. And does it really matter so much. Why the Mount Vesuvius reaction." – I'm not sure it that makes sense, but that's the best way to describe it right now.)

In 2015 we got a call from Canada Revenue.

I was the one who picked up the phone, and I have to admit I laughed when the representative told me we were being reviewed.

I told him his time would be better spent on people who actually made money. We were writers.

He was not amused, asking me a number of questions, including requesting that I pass the phone over to Tony. As I've mentioned, Tony was the financial expert in our household, and for years, I would hand him all of my slips and a tally of income and expenses, in little white envelopes, and he would fill out both of our income tax returns. Apparently, for the first time, he had made an error on mine and, despite the tally I had given him, had failed to report some of my income. I don't know what he and the Revenue agent talked about, though I assume he had made errors on his own as well.

I can't say I was surprised. I still had a ways to go before I would manage to clear up all the unpaid bills I had discovered the year before. I sighed with resignation. Now I would have to take over our income tax, too.

After more missed calls from Mary Beth, I finally told her what was going on — from my perspective at least, since nothing had been confirmed by doctors. Mary Beth could clearly see that he was having memory problems, and all I could add was that the tests showed cognitive gaps. Even as I told her, I was terrified that I had got it all wrong, that I would have to take it all back at a later date and say he was just fine.

I also told Terri one evening when we were out for dinner. Tony's call to her regarding my birthday the previous fall suddenly made sense. He had surprised and upset her by giving her just two days' notice of the party. By then, she had assumed we weren't doing anything and made other plans. Tony also asked her what he should get me for a gift, and when she asked, Well, what does she like? he replied, I don't know. Now she realized that what had seemed like an insensitive comment was not. He really had no idea what I liked.

Terri and I agreed that we should hope for a stroke, that a person could come back from that. Deep down, I no longer believed it. Had I ever? I knew what Alzheimer's looked like.

I had also begun to confide in my neighbour Olga, who had probably figured out what was wrong even before I did. She was not only a former nurse, but had worked at a veteran's hospital where dementia cases were not uncommon. I was having tea with her one day and wondered aloud if the doctors would say that it was Alzheimer's. She replied: Forget about what the doctors think for a minute. What do you think?

She knew that I knew. And under her counsel, I learned to write down my observations, ask questions, and, if need be, copy them into a letter and send that to the doctor so that they would be addressed during an appointment. Doing so would allow me to avoid the awkwardness of asking about these things in front of Tony.

In May I was busy training for an upcoming online mentoring job at Simon Fraser University, as well as working on final edits for my second novel. *Two-Gun & Sun* is full of macabre imagery, of the attempt to find beauty in a place where things are dark and misshapen and frightening. I can see now that these ideas didn't stem solely from my imagination.

I was still teaching writing workshops at UBC. If I didn't like the online format at SFU, at least I would still have that work to fall back on. I was busy, and coming down with a cold, despite the start of what would become a four-month-long heat wave. I was run down.

I have written the following, then cut it from the manuscript, then gone in again to put it back. Always the question: Is there too much me in this? What does this have to do with Tony? If he has the starring role in this story, am I best supporting in a caregiving role? I have said this a story that can't exist without my presence at the keyboard. I'm probably the last person who can determine that for certain, but here goes.

One night I blacked out and came to on the concrete floor, face-first in a pool of blood.

I thought of Tony's fall in the kitchen. I touched finger to nose to make sure I could and that I hadn't had a stroke. God, that was all we needed. I thought of calling an ambulance, but I knew that would throw Tony, or that he might not wake up until the morning and would be in a panic then, wondering where I was. So, I cleaned up the blood and went back to bed. He slept right through it.

First thing in the morning, I took my black eye and swollen nose to the doctor, and she sent me off for appointments to check my heart. I was fine. I have normal-to-low blood pressure, only problematic during a heat wave. It seems the issue was stress. Watching all the changes in Tony and feeling that each time we saw a doctor I was put in the position of trying to convince them, as though I were making it up, and having to go home with him to deal with more problems — well, as Terri later said, no wonder I collapsed.

Tony's doctors didn't know this happened because they'd never asked about my health.

It's a question that should be asked of caregivers more often, and not as the appointment is ending and you have five seconds to answer. Our health should be part of the patient's overall care plan. Without us, appointments can't be booked or attended, medication isn't taken, questions aren't asked.

Years later, I raised this point with my own doctor. She ordered an MRI for me and within two months my brain was scanned. Two months! This had me wondering once more why Tony had to wait so long for his. And again, it showed that my noggin, apparently, is just fine, which is good for all concerned.

Ultimately, that is the reason I've left in this particular incident. I will return to the issue of caregiving in the final chapters. But my role as a writer in this story remains uncertain to me. Do I stay in the background and present the story as I see it from Tony's perspective, or do I disband all attempts to know what he is thinking, give him space to say it himself, and then give myself the space as well?

Early that summer, Tony and his sister Cinda prepared to fly to Toronto to see their sister, Josée, and attend the funeral of her husband, Jerry. He had died after a prolonged struggle with lung cancer.

Their flight was just six months after Tony and I had travelled to Toronto and he had navigated the streets alone. Yet he and Cinda hadn't even left the Vancouver airport before problems began emerging.

Tony lost his boarding pass. He checked all his pockets and bags, and then, instead of going to the desk to report it lost, searched those pockets and bags again, and then again, and yet again, until, finally, in exasperation, Cinda marched over to the desk, where she learned it had been found on the floor and turned in. She kept it for the rest of the trip.

On the plane, she had a long conversation with Tony, and a few minutes later, when she returned from the washroom, she discovered he couldn't recall anything they had just talked about. This shocked her. She'd had that stroke three years before, but her memory was functioning just fine. What was going on with his?

The two have always been close, and seeing for herself some of the signs that I had been mentioning had upset her terribly. They were staying at Chi-Chi's apartment building. Cinda took the spare room and they put Tony in the guest suite. They watched in distress from the elevator as he walked down the hallway, lost, all the doors looking the same to him.

Cinda phoned me in tears, describing what she was seeing. I was not surprised, and, in all honesty, I was almost relieved. It didn't matter how much I repeated what was going on at home. Only personal experience could bring such sudden understanding.

Soon after they returned from Toronto, our year was up, and Tony and I saw the gerontologist again. I described the trip, as well as the year's events.

I mentioned, in particular, that Tony's tendency to repeat a question, or versions of it, had increased. And this was especially true with seemingly small issues. Are you going out? he would ask if I was preparing a dinner just for him. I would tell him all about the event, only to have him ask within the hour, Are you going somewhere? Any actions on my part — ironing an outfit, having a shower, putting on makeup — would elicit the question, Oh, are you going out? Where are you going? Are you going somewhere? Is something happening tonight? And so on.

The gerontologist gave Tony the memory test, and this time his score was lower, around twenty-four or twenty-five — again, I wasn't paying close attention to the numbers then. She prescribed Aricept, looked directly at me and said, We know what this is for.

I nodded, though the doctor didn't know it was the same medication prescribed to my mother for Alzheimer's. I didn't tell her because I was having a hard enough time convincing people, including medical authorities, how bad things were with Tony. I didn't want her thinking I was anticipating problems based on my past experience. All I could do was describe what I was seeing and hope she would draw the appropriate conclusions.

One such incident involved our old washing machine, which often shook out of balance and would hop out of place, jamming the cupboard doors open. I had just put a load of dark laundry in and called Tony because I needed him to shove the heavy machine back in place before I could turn on the water.

He got busy pushing and pulling, and I left the room for a few minutes. When I returned, I was brought to a dead halt.

On every surface — sink, counters, ledge, shower stall, tub, doorknob, medicine cabinet — pieces of black laundry had been draped. It was like an explosion of black, like a scene out of Hitchcock's *The Birds*.

The doctor waited for more.

I said I supposed that Tony thought it could hang to dry instead of going in the dryer, but it had never been washed to begin with. That's why he had helped me. So I could turn on the water.

It was unsettling, I added: the sight of all that black stuff all over.

I wanted to say it wasn't normal, but Tony was sitting right there, and shouldn't such observations come from the doctor?

In a way, it didn't matter. The doctor could be as reluctant as she wanted over naming what was going on — and nowhere on that list of ten warning signs was anything like this mentioned — but I knew there was something was very wrong with Tony's ability to perceive the world around him, even a world as small as our laundry closet.

Since then, I have learned from the gerontologist that this is referred to as a visual or visuospatial problem. The event with the laundry was the result of much the same thing that produced the incident with the cat dishes, I gather. More examples would follow.

Now, she was prescribing Aricept and implying that we knew what this was for.

I waited for her to say the word, *Alzheimer's*, but she didn't, perhaps because, once said, there is no taking it back.

Instead, she said the medication would give me some relief from all the repetition.

The year before, she and the other doctor had mentioned some cognitive gaps in Tony's test responses. Now, she elaborated, calling it mild cognitive impairment, acknowledging that it was a holding-pattern diagnosis. The symptoms could improve, remain the same, or worsen.

I thought through the possibilities. A head injury from, say, a car accident, could improve over time. Cognitive damage from a stroke could be repaired or stabilized if the brain is re-trained to use other neural pathways. I saw that in Cinda. But worsen? That's Alzheimer's.

See you in six months, she said.

I sat up, then. She might not be willing to say the word, but at that point the appointments had always been once a year. Things had worsened.

A brochure distributed by the Alzheimer Society of Canada states, "There is no one single test that can tell if a person has Alzheimer's disease. The diagnosis is made through a systematic assessment which eliminates other possible causes. Until the time when there is a conclusive test, doctors may continue to use the words 'probable Alzheimer's disease.'"

We were not far along in that system, and so we received, instead, a diagnosis of MCI.

John Mann, who had recently gone public about his diagnosis of Alzheimer's disease, put it more succinctly.

I had met him at the gym I joined in an effort to keep in shape to reduce stress. It was there, pulling ropes on one of the kinesis machines, that I found myself working out next to the singer. I said how brave and generous it was of him to go public, and told him that my husband had recently been diagnosed with MCI.

He nodded sympathetically and said, Yeah, they always start with that.

So I knew.

I talked to friends and family who were familiar with what was going on. We compared notes, but I saw more than they did because I lived with Tony, I lived with the complications. I read material and more material, searching for medical evidence of typical clues — those signs, and reports of what I could expect to happen soon, as well as in the future.

This is the true haunting of the disease: we are left alone to draw these conclusions, to sit up at night in the glow of the screen as we search online for terrifying answers no doctor wants to give us.

All the information I found led to one undeniable conclusion. I would put it into words in a notebook that I would share with no one: *My husband is dying, and there is nothing I can do about it.*

This refrain would run through my brain again and again as the pieces of the puzzle began to settle into place, and our likely future took shape.

I wanted confirmation of what I was seeing, but Tony, naturally, wanted the opposite. He wanted hope.

It was like being told in the 17th century that you had indications of leprosy. Your initial thoughts are well that's it, I am going to go through a long horrible period of degradation and will turn into some kind of subhuman, pitiful, creature who is just begging to die but no one will accommodate him.

Probably like a cancer diagnosis once was. "Prepare to die" and that sort of thing, which was common before they had treatments that actually worked.

But, at the same time, I took some solace in my vague knowledge, the advice of the doctor, and my own reading, that this was a possible pre-alzheimer's condition... ONLY, and not an absolute inevitability. Somewhere in the back of my mind, was the rational me pointing out that there are graduations of meaning in the diagnosis that soon become apparent (or are hooks to cling to).

Simply, I didn't trust the overall worries surrounding the diagnosis, or the doctor that gave it. I was smart enough to know that the brain is "elastic" enough that this might not 100-percent be the "end."

So, while I wallowed in pain and fear and worry, I also clung to a light that said "I can beat this thing." Or a the very least keep it to where it is.

# SORRY, YOU CAN'T DRIVE THAT CAR

Initially, Tony was given five milligrams of Aricept per day. I was told that if that dose had little effect after one month, it would be upped to ten milligrams.

The five milligram dose made no difference, so the dosage was increased to ten, and almost immediately the repetition of questions stopped. Tony was keen to keep up with the improvement, and so we began practising the string of words that had stumped him in the last memory test. I told him they would give him a different test next time, but it was the cognitive exercise of remembering that he wanted to practise. Several times a week we went over those words.

In some ways, the prescribing of Aricept made things worse. He could function better, and so the reaction I got from several people, family members included, was that he seemed just fine. He could and still can talk a blue streak, and that ability to articulate was not what the world expects from a person with cognitive problems.

Still, in the fall he hit a slump. My novel *Two-Gun & Sun* was published. I was scheduled to appear in an event at the Vancouver Writers Fest, and the moderator was my friend Jen.

Jen and Mary and I had been friends since forming the writing group SPiN in 2002, and the four of us were planning to go for lunch after. I was looking forward to celebrating. With the cooler weather, my dizzy spells had stopped, and I had managed to finish that novel, throw a launch party, and begin teaching the online course — all the while taking on more and more of the load at home. Looking back, I don't know how I managed to accomplish all that.

Tony was anxious the day of my appearance at the festival. He was having problems with his phone and became desperate to fix it. At the same time, as he was supposed to drive me there, he began fretting about where he was going to park. This had never bothered him before. I had a free ticket waiting for him at the theatre, but at the last minute, he cancelled.

In fact, I asked him, Do you not want to go?

Relief washed over his face, and he asked if I minded if he didn't.

What did I say back? I don't recall. I grabbed my things and rushed to call a cab. I offered the driver a big tip if he could speed and get me there, pronto. Thanks to that cabbie I was on stage on time. It was only after the event ended and Mary, Jen, and I were on our way to lunch that the question was asked, Where's Tony?

There, in the restaurant, my launch done and my festival appearance finished, I told them what was happening. I hate crying in public, but I couldn't seem to get a sentence out without gushing. I knew that if I had told them beforehand I would never have been able to do those events. The diagnosis was still MCI, with only the possibility that things might get worse. What I had experienced that very day, however, didn't offer much hope of improvement. Also, Mary and Jen said they had noted changes in him at the launch, that he seemed confused, and that someone else had wondered if he was drunk.

It was my brother's birthday in December, and as we often did, we picked Tom up to take him for a pub dinner. Tony was driving and on the way there almost ran down a woman at a crosswalk. I insisted on driving back.

That same winter, heading over to a friends' on the North Shore for a party, Tony was cursing and accelerating because it was dark and raining and confusing, and he screeched across six lanes of traffic to reach a gas station. Pamplona came back to me again, and, once more, I drove back.

At the party, among old working buddies, he had seemed fine, but at other events he was sometimes not his usual talkative self.

In explanation of this, he wrote:

> Now, unfortunately, most day to day stuff bores me, tires me out, as does small, meaningless and often repetitive small talk of the type spouted by adults when they get together (Trump's a jerk, work is tough, aren't these house prices crazy, so and so is having such and such troubles, etc., X, who has one track — everybody (except him) is an idiot and crook who is trying to stunt his ambitions, and I'm going to get me a big boat or motor home and —- just live) so I try to avoid them whenever possible, which probably isn't such a good idea because it is isolating (I find them brain numbing, i'd rather talk about something more exciting, like learning). Maybe this MCI is merely a returning of myself to my dreamy, head-in-the-clouds youth, which would be nice. What wouldn't be so nice is

> that it is a form of regression indicative of brain shrink-
> age. Certainly it seems odd to most people, who think you
> should be more "adult" and concentrating on more realis-
> tic things.

The six months had passed and it was a new year, 2016, and time to see the gerontologist again. After hearing about his driving incidents, she suggested he stop driving at night. I told her how the fall had been, and she nodded, and said all indications were that Tony was entering the early stages of Alzheimer's.

The room was suddenly, dizzyingly bright. She had finally said the word. *All indications*, I realize now, sounded just like the *probable* that I had more recently read about in that Alzheimer Society brochure, which had also noted that doctors making this diagnosis are accurate 80 to 90 percent of the time.

I felt hopeful that, finally, we were close to getting answers. When she gave him the usual MoCA, however, he scored a whopping twenty-eight out of thirty. She laughed! What an amazing score.

But, I said, that's the same test you gave him last time. We prac-tised that string of words.

I can say it now, slightly re-arranged to fit with a mnemonic device that I created. I plucked the word *red* from the end of the string and placed it in the middle: Face Velvet Red Daisy Church. Face next to velvet, which I pictured as red, and daisies surround-ing a church. I'll never forget those words. I'll be saying them till the day I die. (The actual order is Face Velvet Church Daisy Red.)

However, the fact that Tony could remember the words, even if they were the same as last time, showed that his brain was some-what capable of remembering, of improving. She said she was still sticking to the diagnosis, but would be happy to be proved wrong. I suppose she was factoring in the 10 to 20 percent of the time when this happened.

She took our application for the Disability Tax Credit — somewhat reluctantly, I thought, but perhaps she felt some doubt, given his high score — and said she would read it over and send it in.

The Disability Tax Credit, once approved, not only opens up eligibility for tax credits in future tax years, but also for refunds on taxes paid in the past, as long as your disability is deemed to have been in place then. In other words, the refund could go back several years and add up to a lot of money, depending on when the diagnosis was dated.

There it was again, that word: *diagnosis.*

Our accountant had given us the form. This was Lorraine, who had worked with me on my father's finances. I had arranged to have her take over the filing of our income tax after those last mistakes Tony made. He said he was glad to be rid of the burden. It would prove to be good timing as this was near the point when Lorraine would discover he had not filed his GST on self-employment earnings since 2012.

For now, Tony was elated by his high score. I was dismayed. At the time, and this is important to remember, he was on Aricept, which boosted his cognitive function and so must have enhanced his test-taking abilities. I wished I could take the doctor home with me and show her what he was like with everyday activities. I knew things would only grow worse, but there was only me to witness them.

And if all indications were that he was heading into early Alzheimer's, why not order an MRI so we could be sure? Tony and I had talked about him getting an MRI, so we could actually see what was happening to his brain, and told the gerontologist we wanted one.

MRIs are expensive, she said, and what would be the point? Tony was already doing what was needed for improved cognitive function. He had quit smoking, cut back on alcohol, improved his diet, and increased his physical and cognitive exercise routine.

I should have said that it was our right to know for certain what was going on in his brain. In that moment, however, I was at a loss for a comeback.

Typically, Tony continued his online search for solutions. If she would be delighted to be proved wrong, he was determined to help her get there.

I spent several days walking and thinking and ruminating and exercising depressing and perhaps even meditating. I turned it over and over again in my mind so that I could see all aspects of it, instead of simply clinging to one possibility — the one we all think of immediately. I poured over every bit of literature I could find on it, online, in the library, or elsewhere.

I watched television shows or movies that discussed the issue (there weren't many, most wanted to stay away from the subject—bad juju). I think one movie we watched was "Still Alice", which, even then, I realized was an overly dramatized situation — a storyline that cut out all the subtleties and alternatives and went in a straight line to the worst possible conclusion. Hey, I'm enough of a writer to know that all stories don't have to end in the most dramatic way, and that the vast majority are far less exciting and definitive, but probably more accurate. Still, it was frightening. Good storytelling can be powerful.

But I continued researching the brain and how it works, etc. and discovered the concept of brain plasticity which had just been discovered. It holds that the brain can, essentially, repair itself — perhaps not to a no-alzheimer's indication degree, but to something acceptable. At least, I reasoned, (Hah, bad joke), with exercise, the right nutrition, etc. I could repair my brain to the point where I was somewhat normal, if not perfect.

So, I plunged into learning as much as I could about plasticity, nutrition, etc. — an exercise, I believe, that helped as much as any other in that I had something to focus on besides my own problems, in that it gave me a purpose. Of course there were dark moments along the way, many lingering worries, like how was I ever going to please my dead mother's admonitions to make money, be perfect, and all the other stuff I had been dealing with most of my life.

One bonus of the diagnosis was that I could throw all that past away; I could start brand new, today was day one of the rest of my life, and other cliches. Also, that I could now design my life to be the way I wanted it to be. Yes, I had money worries, and yes, you (June) wouldn't be happy about all the changes — no one likes to see the familiar disappear overnight, and yes there would be a long period where friends, and even myself, would balk at the changes and try for the familiar.

But I was going to do it, dammit. My life had changed and I was going to accept that change, despite the dislikes or complaints of others and of those nattering voices that we all carry in our heads, despite the prospect of failure and looming, drooling senility, despite lack of money and the constant (societal and personal) emphasis on spending (or not) it and resulting depression, despite the likely disappearance of "friends", and the corollary disappearance of my own sense of place in the world.

Life, as I knew it, was over to some degree, and I would go with that change; I would live it as best I could. I would do many of the things I always wanted to do, pursue many of the pursuits I had dreamed of, etc. This didn't mean running off to Tahiti or something ridiculous as that. Instead it simply meant that I would retreat into the person I once was: Adventurous in that I was always willing to try new things, dreamy and thoughtful, a learner, a "try-er" — essentially, an explorer.

Senility and Madness was not a hard and fast inevitability, but it was a possibility and I had to accept that it might come. So there was no time to lose.

# REJECTED BY THE GOVERNMENT, OR, YOU SEEM JUST FINE TO US

Within two months, Tony was doing anything but proving the doctor wrong.

We were having changes made to one bathroom, which included, at long last, a new washer/dryer set that wouldn't hop out of the closet, and a new, second half-bathroom. Our neighbour Tina has an eye for design and helped draw up the plans.

The following year, Tony would be asked to explain the need for this powder room in a letter to the government that would give us a home accessibility grant.

Aricept is well-known for its effects on the gastro-intestinal system, and when the urge to go strikes, Tony wrote, I need to get to the facilities immediately and it had better not be already occupied. Our solution after enduring this for almost a year was to install a second toilet.

In fact, I wrote it and he signed it, because, while the words came from Tony, the actual act of sitting down to compose it and then email it to Lorraine as an attachment proved too much. The construction was disruptive, and likely was hard on his cognitive function, as was the natural progression of the disease.

Our neighbour Richard had been growing ill with cancer. The usual Friday evening get-togethers he and Tony shared were now taking place only once every two weeks. The jokester neighbour who once "borrowed" a pair of my black fishnet pantyhose, then returned in a raincoat to flash me, wearing only the pantyhose and a black codpiece — yes, I shrieked — had become gaunt and weak.

He had always enjoyed cooking, but now had to ask Tony to take on some of the meals, giving him specific instructions. Tony was never a fancy cook and did his best, and now he had forgetfulness compromising things further.

One night, on a hunch that things might not be right, I came back early from a dinner with Terri. We walked into the apartment and into a wall of heat. Under Richard's instructions, Tony had dashed over to our place to grill something in the oven. He had not only forgotten to turn the oven off, but had also neglected to close the oven door. Again, I pictured a breeze from an open window sending a piece of paper wafting into the oven and starting a fire. Or the curious cats, smelling meat ...

I knew I would have to talk to Richard soon. It happened after he asked Tony to drive him to a medical appointment out at UBC. Although the gerontologist had recommended that Tony not drive at night, she said that driving in the day should still be fine. She warned us this could change, though, and it certainly did. Tony drove Richard to UBC without incident, but it clearly fatigued him to drive all that way. I didn't want either of them risking such a drive again. I pulled Richard aside to explain some of what was going on. He didn't say anything, and I wasn't sure if he had understood me. As it turns out, he had. I would learn much later that he had told his partner Manny I was in for a tough time.

At any rate, I was glad I had spoken up then, because Tony began to grow confused behind the wheel, even in daylight hours.

One time, he was driving along Grandview Highway and kept asking, Where's Grandview Highway? When I assured him we were on Grandview Highway, he said it didn't look the same. We were passing by Trout Lake, which has not changed.

Another time, he was pulling out of a shop where we had just picked up bathroom tiles for the renovation. He couldn't seem to recognize the concrete island that divided the two directions of traffic on busy Willingdon Avenue, and wanted to turn left into the oncoming traffic, as that was the direction we had come from. It would have meant certain injury, if not death. I shouted No, and several times had to yell the direction, turn right, turn right, in order to convince him.

The final incident, the one that persuaded me that Tony was no longer able to drive, took place two blocks from our place, where we needed to turn right onto Rupert Street to head south. He kept trying to turn left, and when I asked why, he said, I need to find Rupert Street. I told him this was Rupert Street, but when that didn't compute, I said, Pull over. He did, and I got behind the wheel, but he was furious with me.

Only now, in writing this, do I realize that two of the incidents involved a persistence in wanting to turn left, as though something in his brain had shorted out, stopping his ability to turn right.

Back then, and once home, I tried to explain my concerns about his driving at all in the same way that the gerontologist had first explained the need to stop driving at night. You might be fine 95 percent of the time, I repeated, but it's that 5 percent that's a concern. You could injure yourself or someone else.

He was angry, though. This was a loss of control, of something he had been very good at. He used to drive a sports car, after all, and a motorcycle.

I don't know what I said next — the memory of it is consumed in the words that followed. He said, If you talk to me like that again, I'll punch you in the face.

I didn't cry. I was numb. He has never hit me, I should add here, but the Tony I knew, in that moment at least, had vanished, and I began the long process of grieving for the life we had once had and the future we had planned but would never see.

He has no recollection of saying those specific words to me, but acknowledges the frustration he often feels.

> I think "what's with you treating me like a recalcitrant child? Who do you think you are anyway to be giving me shit or ordering me around?" I think I may have even voiced versions of this sometimes, for which I now apologize. I do have a temper, just as you do — it comes with the emotional being. But when two people with tempers clash, it's fireworks — and not always of the good kind.

It would be worthwhile to show more examples of what might have been going on in his head, but by virtue of the disease, his responses can be random and sporadic, and are not always in sync with this timeline.

Again, the renovation added to the general stress level, and on top of this, his sister Josée was coming out for a visit. He was anxious, saying that he didn't want to look stupid in front of her.

Around this time, he had a falling out with someone as a result of a joke he made about that person getting support from a spouse. It fell flat. He meant emotional support but the person Tony was talking to thought that Tony meant financial support. Tony later apologized, though a person with dementia can't be faulted for an awkward comment. The rest of us have to make the adjustment. It could be this other person was unaware of the full extent of Tony's impairment. We were still without a formal diagnosis. My mother once surprised me by loudly remarking that her nurse considered herself King Shit. This, from someone who never swore. I tried to quiet her and say that wasn't nice. Okay, she said, smirking, Queen Shit, then. In Tony's case, the offence was unintentional, but only the passage of time mended the rift.

Depression clouded his mind.

He accidentally disconnected the hose at the back of our new washer, and water seeped into our downstairs neighbours' closet. I offered to have it repainted, but Tim and Judith very kindly said it didn't matter. No one could see it.

Their kindness would be called upon again when Tony went for a bike ride, and tied his bag of personal effects to the back of his bike with a length of string. It fell off somewhere along the bike route, and he rode back and forth, frantically, trying to find where it had dropped. It was growing dark, and I was preparing to call the police, wondering how I would even phrase it: Indications are he is heading into Alzheimer's ... but not confirmed, so, no, he wears no MedicAlert tag, what would it say? Indications are ...?

He walked through the door then, looking drained. He hadn't phoned me because his phone was in the bag, along with wallet and keys. That meant that any thief that found it not only had his money and bank cards but also his address and the keys to access our building.

Everyone has lost their keys or wallet at some point in their lives, true. But when it happens, they take action. Tony didn't know what to do.

Together, we cancelled all the cards and the phone. I got in touch with Tim and Olga and we alerted the building. By morning, I had arranged to have the locks changed and would be in charge of getting new building keys to all — not just fellow-residents but also all the companies that conduct work in the building. Phone, hydro, cable, plumbers.… It took several days and cost us several hundred dollars, and, of course, Tony could not take on any of this. There were too many steps involved, too many things to remember, and there was too little money in his bank account.

I was reaching overload. I was about to complete a full school year mentoring students in the online writing program. With the help of Garth and Joni, who had corrected some of the online glitches that had plagued my progress, the last several months had run smoothly. Still, other mentors had begun experiencing technical problems, so the program was going to switch to an upgraded system — a new one for me to learn. I made the tough decision to not return in the fall. Given all I was facing with Tony, who had, at times, dismantled my computer equipment when he didn't recognize it as his, I was glad I had, and by the fall I had switched virtual for real classrooms.

I had no sooner finished reshuffling our money to finally pay off the last of the household debt, than we got a call from the bank.

At first I thought they might be calling in the loan, but the accounts manager was simply advising us that payments hadn't been made. I asked for details and he wouldn't elaborate. Ah, I thought. They can involve me only so far. I co-signed, but it's Tony's account.

The POA papers were folded and in my shoulder bag when I took Tony up to the bank and sat with another manager to discuss the line of credit. With him beside me, she seemed quite willing to do so. I learned that Tony had not only not made any payments, but had withdrawn several thousand to pay his annual tax bill.

We had hit that magic moment in finances where interest and other fees along with withdrawals began a snowball effect. The debt had swelled to frightening proportions.

I suggested that from then on the only activity with the line of credit be payments. No more withdrawals.

Except for his annual income tax payments, she suggested, since this is a business loan.

I looked at Tony and took a deep breath, not knowing what he would say to my answer.

No, I told her, not even for that.

I added that a small payment should go automatically from our joint account to the line of credit each month to ensure that some money always went in and that the debt did not increase. This made both of them happy, and we set that up on the spot. I did this without having to haul the POA out of my bag, which was good, since without a doctor's letter, this bank would not have considered it valid.

I would later learn from other caregivers that the tactic I used at the bank is called creative fibbing. I had no legal right to make the changes to the payments, but because I brought Tony with me and said something that pleased both of them, no one objected.

Many times since then Tony has asked how we are supposed to pay his taxes now. I explain that we will have to withdraw from his savings to do so. He has said repeatedly that he worries about that amount being depleted, and repeatedly I have answered that depleting the savings is better than increasing the debt. Then, in a turnabout that startles me each time, he confuses the debt for the savings, and I see anew how the numbers he once knew so well had meshed together to become a digital gibberish to him.

Around this time, I joined the Alzheimer's Society's Young Onset Spouses Support Group, not even sure if my spouse definitely had Alzheimer's or if he could really be considered someone with young-onset, given that he was now in his mid-sixties. The society representative said to me that if he had it now then he had likely been showing signs for many years. I burst into tears to hear such welcome understanding.

Yet another bank incident wrapped up 2016. Tony had neglected to deposit a cheque, and so I said I would drive him to the bank to make sure it happened. He got out of the car and, instead of opening the glass door to the bank, began running his fingernails around the edges of the window, as though it was a portal into the bank, or ATM. He finally gave up and returned to the car. As he explains it:

> My memory isn't instant for some things: at this age the hard drive is getting full, as they say. But that's common to all, and so, for the most part it's not affecting me that much.
>
> But sometimes it is. I will be in the middle of saying something, and can't find the right word, or recall a conversation — which, I admit, happens quite often (largely because I wasn't that interested, I think). Other times I will be off in dream land or something and not really be aware of much at all. But I've always been like that at times, except for when I was working and then really focused.
>
> And sometimes, it's starker and more obvious. The most recent, and concerning to you, I think involved our visit to the bank. So let me paint the picture.
>
> We were in the car, going somewhere, and as often occurs when I'm in the car and not driving, I wasn't really "there" — just drifting, not really thinking of anything, just giving my brain a rest, so to speak. However, we might have had some kind of minor argument earlier and that was still on my mind.

We had to stop at the bank to use the automatic teller machine to get some cash, and we pulled up, I hopped out of the car to go in, and .... stopped. The door was locked, it was dark inside and outside — raining I believe — and it all looked so .....unfamiliar (I am more used to seeing it in the daytime." This quick moment of confusion has happened before when it is dark — I'm much affected by light and the lack of it — and I couldn't focus. For a few seconds I didn't understand where I was, didn't recognize any of the familiar markers that said "door", "window", etc.

However, there was a big, lighted, poster of a bank on the window and I was drawn to it, immediately looking for the knob or pull to open the door. But I couldn't find it, and so started feeling around the poster for the entrance.

That is what concerned you, I think, and frankly concerned me as well. Of course, I quicky realized what I was doing, and moved to the real door which was beside it, just as you were saying something about it — and showing much concern about the strangeness of my actions.

Admittedly, I was shaken. That had never happened to me before. This was especially true when you asked me about it as I got in the car. All I could say was that I couldn't see it.

This was true, of course. I couldn't. I seem to be having increasing difficulties seeing in the darkness — which in Vancouver is literally most of the time, at this time of year, because the rain and cloud of Winter is seeming- ly ever present. I have noticed that I am often confused at night time when familiar "markers" are hidden. That is why, when I am walking in unfamiliar territory at night, I often get confused as to where I am. Whether this began with my condition, or before, I'm not sure. I think it was always there — I remember, when I was young, having some awareness that everything looked different at night and that, frankly, without my glasses, I was almost blind if it was dark and I wasn't on some well-travelled route that had familiar markers (that I could see).

But this was somewhat different than that. There was some light. It shouldn't have been unfamiliar — I had been there many times — but somehow it was.

I think I described it as "like when you're listening to music or something else and there's a blip in the recording and for that moment you're completely confused." Except with a blip in a recording, it's over in a second or two. In my case, it wasn't over in a second or two (although that used to be the case). It continued for a minute or two.

And that, I think, was what frightened us both: That moment of utter confusion.

The year ended with the departure of Cinda and Godwin for a new home in Toronto, and the death of our friend and neighbour Richard. Tony believes strongly that there is a connection between depression and cognitive decline, and he worked hard to fight this. Still, I could see him floundering in the months that followed.

# THE SECRET OF YOUR DISEASE

The year 2017 was a strange one. We were moving through mud, each step forward a hard slog. It was a half-life, in which the disease, with no written or formal diagnosis, kept us financially troubled and emotionally stifled — in a silent grief in which we were alone to contemplate this uncertain future.

According to the government, Tony did not have a cognitive disability. Our application for the Disability Tax Credit, initially filed in 2016, was rejected. And the financial issues continued.

Early in the year, we had to cash in RRSPs to pay for our share of roof construction on the apartment building. To make it easier on us at income tax time, the investment company suggested Tony write a series of letters dated a day apart requesting small sums on each. Tony grew increasingly agitated and angry over the complications involved, so I wrote them out and forwarded them to him to sign and send.

Next, he was instructed to send a void cheque so that these amounts could be sent to our bank account and from there to the roof fund. He was furious because he couldn't find the cord to the scanner. To calm him down, I followed the bank's suggestion that we take a picture of the void cheque and then email it. I told the bank I was using my phone as he was having trouble with his, which was a creative white lie-and-a-half. They only agreed to me sending it because he had already begun the process.

We saw the gerontologist shortly after this, at which time we explained that the application for the Disability Tax Credit had been rejected and asked her if she could try again.

Our accountant had taken one look at that first attempt in 2016 and told us we wouldn't get it, though she sent it on to the government anyway. I had supplied some of my own anecdotal evidence, as someone else I know had similarly done and to positive effect, but Lorraine said that made the application far too detailed. Simple is what they were after.

Further, the application normally requires two categories of impairment and, when the doctor went through the lists of activities of daily living (ADLs), she had to check no for such things as, Does he need assistance bathing, getting dressed, using the washroom, or eating food?

The medical comments on page 5 had said: "The patient can manage his ADLs but he needs support from his family for ADLs as outlined. He can no longer work and is restricted in how much he can contribute to the family — can't cook safely or do financial transactions."

It sounded good to me, but what it was missing, I would learn, was the all-important word that would make all other categories of ADLs unnecessary: *dementia*, or *Alzheimer's*.

Lorraine said this was not unusual. Many doctors do not understand how this tax application works. In fact, much later another specialist assured me that Tony wouldn't qualify because he was retired, mistaking the Disability Tax Credit for a worker's disability pension.

It was an important lesson for us. Why would the doctors know better? They were cognitive and brain specialists, not tax specialists.

Lorraine *was* a tax specialist, and kindly offered to explain to the doctor what was needed so that we could re-apply.

We gave the gerontologist the new application form and told her she would be hearing from Lorraine. In the meantime, I also asked if she would please enact the power of attorney, telling her what had happened with the RRSPs, and how much easier it would have been had I been able to do it all on my own. A letter activating the POA would have to come from her.

She told me that she had to decline my request, at least for the time being, citing the need to allow Tony to maintain his dignity and the need for him to feel in control after having lost so much. I might have been angry if not for what I had learned back when I was taking my mother to appointments. The doctor's main concern, I reminded myself, is the patient, and that wasn't me. But I was disappointed, and so tired.

During this time, Tony was becoming repetitive again, which raised the question of whether the Aricept still worked. There is some belief that after a while its effectiveness wears off. This hasn't been the case for Tony. A number of times, when he became visibly confused or suddenly misplaced things more than usual, I would find, when I checked his pills, that he had forgotten to take them, or had dropped one on the floor. So, for him, at least, the medication did make a difference, and still does, though eventually the disease will progress despite the pills.

There were many people, neighbours and family members, as well as acquaintances and editors who worked with Tony and didn't know about his condition. This was either because he didn't tell them, or they weren't around him enough to detect a difference. I've always wondered why his editors didn't notice, but no one except me knew how much longer his written pieces were taking, and I suppose any errors or missed deadlines were dismissed as being typical of a busy journalist. As for others in our lives, some of those who did know what was going on still committed the outrageous sin of telling me that he looked just fine when they saw him. Of course he did, I wanted to tell them, because when they saw him, all he did was eat dinner and chat pleasantly. Often, I would look at Tony and think that this year was being defined by what I called "the secret of your disease."

One time, though, Tony accidentally let the secret out. We had been to see the documentary *Spirit Unforgettable* with our friends Ted and Fiona. This is a film about the singer John Mann, and his diagnosis of Alzheimer's. I was surprised that Tony wanted to go, and his assurance that he did implied he wanted to see the facts to prove to himself there was no danger of him developing the disease.

Ted and Fiona had to leave early but we stayed for the discussion. The man who had worked out next to me at the gym over a year ago now walked gingerly onto the stage with the help of his band members.

After the talk, Tony headed for the exit doors, where we ran into old friends Glen and Kathy, who suggested we go for dinner. Glen had worked in the newsroom with Tony, and in his current role was an arts reviewer. Through his work, he was acquainted with John Mann and the band. He and Kathy had even been invited to one of the after-film parties. They were surprised to see us at the film, and asked us about our connection to Mann. Tony replied that he'd been to see one of the doctors in the film, and that his score on the test was a few points higher than John's. Glen looked momentarily puzzled, then turned to me. There was no sense in pretending, now, so I said I knew John Mann from the gym, and added that his wife, the actor Jill Daum, went to the same support group I attended.

There were a couple of private moments in the evening when I could elaborate. Glen had pulled me aside to ask if Tony was okay. Emboldened by both Tony's remark and all of the similarities between Tony and John that I saw in the film, I said no, that we were likely looking at the same thing John had.

Early cherry trees were in blossom in the west end that February of 2017 as we moved ourselves and our cats into The Sylvia Hotel. We were there for three weeks in anticipation of noisy roof work overhead. It was a significant period for a couple of reasons.

One reason was that because we were staying close by, Tony tried out an organization called Paul's Club. This came about because we had met club organizers Nita and Michael Levy in a coffee shop. We have friends in common, so I knew about Paul's Club — an organization that runs an adult social and recreational program for those who are still fit but living with young-onset dementia. While chatting with Michael and Nita, Tony forgot his grandchildren's names. It was clear that he was an ideal candidate for the club. They invited him to try it out, and he agreed, liking the sounds of a group that went for regular walks.

I took him over that first day and when I picked him up later he was furious. He suspected everyone there had dementia, except him. I had also noticed that some were visibly affected, and I called Nita with our concerns. She was wonderful, taking the time to carefully explain. I gather that many look like Tony when they first arrive, but as the disease progresses, they change. It was a sobering realization.

To my surprise, Tony agreed to give it another try, and he has been attending ever since. I know he enjoys it there because every summer when we attend the annual baseball fundraiser, Tony leaves me in the dust as soon as he spots his pals from the club. It has been a relief to witness that.

The other reason our stay at The Sylvia was significant was that during one of our beach strolls (how unlike the East Vancouver neighbourhood where we live), we came up with the idea of writing this book.

In my first email to Tony, I wrote: I'm sending this email because you and I talked about putting together a book, and emails back and forth might prove a useful format. Okay, they'll also serve as reminders. You suggested the title *Four Umbrellas*.

I would send him emails and then, when I didn't get a response within a few days, I'd send him reminders, telling him that he hadn't responded to my initial email. The reminders often numbered three or more for each response I would get from Tony. As well, he quickly forgot that the title was his idea, and a year later when the subject came up again, he wrote:

> You just pointed out that the title Four Umbrellas was my idea.....which astonished me. Really? was my reaction. Whatever did I mean by that?
>
> Was I comparing the worldview of my brain to a beach scene where my thinking was divided off into categories in which a lot of material was organized, or hidden or, eventually lost?
>
> Was I being mystical? Somehow thinking in Zen, or other Eastern terms from long ago (which I had just read about in my general travels through ancient writing about the mind?)

Or was I thinking literally, that four umbrellas represent-
ed shelter from the rain (or sun), at a beach or somewhere — shelter from the "attack" on ideas, concepts,
or thoughts that spring from my brain. Or a method of
sorting and storing creativity that indicated a diminishing
of my cognitive/creative abilities? Or, to elaborate on an
earlier point, was I describing the way the brain works, i.e.
putting various information and thoughts under certain
categories (ie. umbrellas)?

Or was it something else entirely? Maybe the four uses of
the brain — recording, analysis, understanding, retrieval?,
I confess, I really can't remember ..... which is a classic
case of what I am continually talking about. I come up
with an idea, and it eventually disappears, maybe not in
an hour, or even a day, but soon after. Then through time,
it disappears completely.

Most recently, that is becoming within minutes, which
seems to indcate a lack of attention, (over which I mentally beat myself up constantly).

I have been pretty fuzzy lately, and especially forgetful —
it's as if I don't hear things, or they don't register in my
brain. More than likely, I hear them, but I'm too busy thinking about repercussions, or what I'm going to say, or how
someone looked, or how this reminds me of something
completely unrelated, to remember them. This isn't new,
but it is far worse than when I was simply absent- minded.
It's as if I didn't fully hear, or see, or understand.

*Four Umbrellas* is not a title with some particular literary or
spiritual significance, of course; it is a literal reference to four umbrellas Tony crammed into his suitcase for our stay at The Sylvia.

However, it does possess, as well, a figurative quality, alluding to the act of repetition, which Tony saw as a classic symptom of cognitive impairment. Specifically, it's a noted symptom of Alzheimer's. At the time he suggested the title, however, Tony hadn't yet come to grips with that latter possibility.

For expediency, he and I often abbreviated the title to its initials. I remarked on the startling sight of *F.U.* on the page, and asked if that was the result of the devious old journo in him. He took a close look at the page and sat back, immensely pleased with it and himself. It reminds me of the term he and his news buddies used to describe the savings each would amass to get them out of the newsroom: the *Fuck You Fund*.

# PART THREE

# THINGS REALLY
# FALL APART

# HURRY UP AND WAIT

During the previous fall, in 2016, we had been to see Tony's new family doctor. His old doctor had retired, a fact we had only discovered in trying to book the appointment, and so we had to re-explain his situation. I asked for a referral to a neurologist so we could finally get an MRI, but the doctor was not convinced Tony needed one. On a second visit, things had changed. He asked Tony a few basic questions about our family and our home, and each time Tony was stumped and turned to me for the answer.

We got the referral, and in April 2017, over six years after Tony's fall in the kitchen, we headed out on our first visit to the Djavad Mowafaghian Centre for Brain Health at UBC Hospital.

As I mentioned in the introduction, Tony scored twenty-six out of thirty on the memory test, and conversed well with the neurologist. This is when I heard that the problem could be normal aging.

I truly wondered: Did no one believe us?

The neurologist wasn't finished, though. For someone like an assembly-line worker, he explained, the short test is just fine, but Tony had been a journalist. That was a career that required knowledge and quick-thinking, in addition to a facility with language. He needed a more intensive test.

My mother had worked on an assembly line, and she was very bright, but I got what he meant. He ordered up a SPECT scan, a single-proton emission computed tomograph, which shows how blood is circulating in the brain, as well as the long-awaited MRI, and a day-long series of neuropsychological tests.

The MRI was just one month later, but when we made the long trip back out to UBC, we discovered that, due to a clerical error, Tony was not in the system.

We received an apologetic phone call the next day. The MRI would have to be re-booked.

It was disappointing, and the wait, we were told, would be several months.

Meanwhile, our accountant Lorraine had, as promised, explained to the gerontologist what was needed for the Disability Tax Credit: that magic word, *dementia*. This gave us another go at the application, and I wanted to know how Tony felt about it all. As mentioned, a response from Tony often required several reminders, as the following exchange shows.

June 1, 2017

I didn't get a reply from you so this is just another nudge. We went to see our accountant so you could sign the disability tax credit form that she had the gerontologist fill out. We've been waiting a long time for that. On the form the doctor used the term "dementia." We've also been waiting a long time for a diagnosis in writing, which is important for all those forms, but how did it feel to read that? Does it change anything for you?

June 26, 2017

This is nudge number three.

I wondered if the diagnosis on the Disability Tax Credit form was the reason for your silence, but you have been free about your feelings when we talk. And then I wondered if perhaps I should tell you how I felt to see the diagnosis. That might stimulate discussion.

So here goes. At first, I was pleased to see it in black and white. Neither of us were convinced when the neurologist said your memory problems could be simply the result of natural aging. After we saw the diagnosis and you signed it, I immediately asked for a photocopy. I realized that every concern I'd had was now confirmed, and if someone were to say to me that you seemed just fine, I could say to myself or to that person — and not doubt myself all over again — yes, he has days when he does seem just fine. It has been hard to see the gaps in your memory and sometimes in day-to-day functions, and repeat these concerns to others, to doctors, and hear replies such as, "Is it just you who notices this?" They are looking for confirmation from others, true, but the implication is that I am imagining things.

And how can we get help if I'm the only one noticing there's a problem? Now I see a way forward, the possibility of financial help, which we badly need.

But there is also a finality to a diagnosis. I stared at the word "dementia," felt my guts clench, my lungs tighten. Okay, I thought: this is real.

The very fact that I need no longer doubt myself also means I can no longer entertain rosy fantasies of, say, moving to another country. We can't be off the Canadian medical grid for long. You remarked after one of our many trips out to the UBC Centre for Brain Health that we can no longer think about moving even to Nelson, BC. That sort of facility is not available there. We probably wouldn't have moved there anyway, but now we can't, and there is a tangible different between "wouldn't have" and "can't."

I have heard that for some couples there comes a certain sense of peace in this situation. They aren't out there climbing the corporate ladder, or jet-setting around the world, or leading an active social life. They spend more time at home and learn to enjoy barbecuing a simple meal or watching a funny movie together. And that does sound like us. We have to take things day by day because our future is more uncertain than it was the day before the diagnosis. Our lives have become somewhat smaller with it. The gods have been generous this summer, giving us two weddings to attend, both out of town, a couple of days each of merriment and celebration, and good people to share that joy with. And if summer is as far ahead as we should be looking, then I, too, feel a certain sense of peace. But you know me. I'm a planner.

Well, that's my take so far. Over to you.

June 26, 2017

Well, lots to chew on here. Maybe because we left it for a while and so there was more to ... uh... chew on.

Anyway, jokes aside, I can probably answer all your questions with a simple sentence and a reference to your description of how we now live.

Essentially, I have grown to accept it all. I recognize I have a problem, that it is now part of my personality (and life), and that, while I can continue to work on it, try to improve it, or at the least, keep it to where it is, it will govern things.

I am no longer in denial — how could I be after all those tests and several episodes where I was "fuzzy" or confused? There have been times where I am simply forgetful — "Did I say that?", "Did I do that?" — to where I am .... well, I don't know what I am... out of it, I guess is the best way to describe it. Confused, like the guy in the movie after an explosion or something, who is just walking around in a daze. I guess that's me occasionally, in a daze.

Inside, it's like I just can't focus on what's going on, or can't hear what people are saying.Whatever, the information just isn't getting through, and I have to work to understand — note to self: practice focusing again. Other times, it's just slowness — especially when you say something or something else is going on, and I know it, but am taking time to digest it. In those cases, it's not so much a mental problem, as a  personal one — I just don't want to think about what you're saying, so have to yank my focus from whatever to what you mentioned (when I really don't care). That, I think, might be more about "tuning out", like you see in the TV shows, etc, than MCI.

Another problem I am noticing is that I am committing more errors lately. For example, my writing has become atrocious, partly because I am "somewhere else", i.e. MCI dreaming, or partly because I am in too much of a hurry. I can no longer write quickly like I one did and still be legible. I now have to concentrate on making the letters right. Also, my spelling is becoming worse. There was a time when I was an almost perfect speller, but now, every few words, there is a ridiculously bad spelling error, or something left out completely. Again, this might be me trying to maintain the same speed I once had when I can't "do" it. So again, I believe it can be corrected if I simply slow down (which isn't always easy.

This need to slow down shows up in other places — often when you're talking with me and want something. I take time to think, which bothers you, or I just answer whatever pops into my head (usually anger) which also bothers you. Whichever, it's frustrating for both of us. Needing time to form thoughts or answers is a sign that the brain is slowing down.

Of course, I also have to question how much of this is MCI, and how much is simply aging, as well as poor hearing. I'm not sure, but I think the "solution" — or at least one remedy — might be just to practice concentration more. Many times, my lack of focus is because I am thinking about something else and am unable to "multi-task" in a sense.

Anyway, enough of the woes; what are the effects?

Well, in a strange way, I feel more peaceful than ever. I rarely worry any more, largely because I realize that not much matters one way or another. I think that is a common situation when one gets older, but I might be getting it a bit early. Some people I know "rage,rage against the dying of the light" until well into their 70's. My rage seems to be fading in my 60's

Is that a bad thing. I don't believe so any more. Increasingly, my viewpoint of most things is "Que sera, sera" - what ever will be, will be. If someone's unhappy, I feel for them, but I don't feel like them — I sympathize from a distance. If they are angry, I let it roll off me; if the are happy, I bask in the glow, if they are successful, I am happy for them, instead of being jealous (although I do get the occasional twinge of "I shoulda/coulda, done that, but it's too late."

I guess that's my main feeling now — I realize it is, in many ways, too late. This, I believe, is a feeling experienced by most people as they age, but I never thought it would affect me. I always though I would rage rage against the dying of the light forever. (of course, those who insist on that, like Dylan Thomas, etc, lived by the "live fast, die young and have a good-looking corpse" attitude — I know I did when I was young.

I don't think I'm unique in all this — and suspect it is a common feeling among people my age or those, who like me are getting a strong glimpse of the "long slow fade", although my glimpse seems to be a little more clear than most others'.

Or maybe not. Maybe I'm just husbanding my resources, concentrating my troops, honing my focus, and ignoring the irrelevant. I'm trying to think that is it, that I can still do something about this by "retraining" myself — with a modicum of self-acceptance and care at the same time.

But I am off track. The simple truth is that there is a kind of peace growing in me, an acceptance of what is. It doesn't mean I won't keep trying, but I won't be upset if it doesn't work, or if trying becomes to difficult.

Simply, it is what it is. I have a condition. It exists. I have to accept it and deal with it. There is no use or point in crying over spilled milk. Shit happens, and other cliches.

It certainly makes things easier.

At home, things progressed as expected, as they still do. These are typical examples.

Tony can't recall what he had for lunch.

I find lettuce in the freezer, dental floss in the fridge.

The fried rice ends up in the cupboard, as does a block of cheese, each going undiscovered for days. The incidents of spoiled food is too long to list here, but it plays havoc on our budget.

Tony goes to the store and leaves his wallet there.

In the evenings when we watch a movie or episodes of a series, he struggles to follow complicated plots or flashbacks.

He takes one of the cats upstairs for fresh air on the roof deck, and forgets him there.

He loses jackets and hats.

I find a piece of paper on which he has tried to determine his age by subtracting his birthdate from 2017, and winds up with 208 years old.

Sometimes, that seems exactly right.

All this time, Tony was still writing his column for the *Financial Post*, and having more difficulty with it. No wonder. I am amazed now that he could write it at all. Frequently, the copy was sent back with errors to fix. I asked him if he was printing a hard copy? That would be a good way to catch those errors. But no, he persisted in sending directly from the screen. That might work for some, but clearly not for him.

He missed deadlines, and always scrambled to send in late copy. He told me that one time an editor expressed frustration with him, noting that while they had had a long discussion about a new deadline, he had forgotten anyway.

Sometimes, he sent the wrong draft.

In April, the very same month we first went to the UBC Centre for Brain Health and an MRI scan of his brain had been ordered, Tony had written an article for the *Financial Post* on generational change in traditional industries. Written in the crisp business style that was typical of Tony's work for the *Post*, it also includes an error, the repetition of a line, slightly re-phrased the second time. Interestingly, the editor missed it as well. When I looked two years later, the mistake was still there. But this just was not like Tony. He used to run the rewrite desk, and had a sharp eye for such glitches.

Things were falling apart in unexpected ways, from the important to the mundane. One morning, I was in a hurry to make breakfast. Where was the toaster? Tony had used it last.

We searched in the usual spots. All the cupboards. The hallway closet. No. I tried the freezer, under the sink. No, no. I stood back, then stepped forward, pulling open the oven door in an aha moment, then the drawer beneath the oven, the shelf beside it. No, no, no to each of these.

At last, I yanked open the microwave oven door and there it was, squeezed tightly into the space, as precisely as only a former engineering student could have imagined it would fit.

I could not get over the significance of this image. Somewhere in the recesses of his mind the creative challenge of structure had overtaken the present need to do something practical: put away the toaster in a place where we could find it. He clearly hadn't thought that putting it there would send sparks flying at the push of a button. I thought of what he had written recently about his university days, and his tendency to embrace the creative, unprofitable aspects of life:

I remember oce in university, the don of my residence — an English guy studying chemistry and destined for some high job in a chemical plant — commenced during a drinking session to analyze all of us younger students. When it was my turn, he commented that I was a "philosopher." I found this exciting and spot on, I suddenly believed that was exactly right. Then he said, "you know what philosophers eat for breakfast? Nothing!

I was devastated. Not only was it cruel, it was true — philosophers made no money, and money was a big thing in my life — partly because I had none, and partly because my mother was constantly harping on it, in turn, making me think that it was completely disgusting and venal, something the stupid people cared about — more clothes, more cars, better houses, etc.

I asked Tony recently if he had switched from engineering to liberal arts before or after this discussion. He said it was before.

As I reached up for the toaster, I was noting that this was another example of his visuospatial impairment. It takes brains to eyeball a space and calculate what will fit into that space, but these two items were as impractical a coupling as keys or wristwatch left in the sugar bowl, the image often used as a typical warning sign of Alzheimer's.

# A SPECTACULAR FLAMEOUT

Memories spring up unexpectedly. They move sideways, they curl and twist, looping back on themselves, a switchback of recollections that cut a crooked path to the past. Much as I try to order my memories, I no sooner line them up and prepare to move forward than out pops another early sign that I had missed, yanking me back yet again. And this from the spouse who, so far at least, has no cognitive issues.

I am walking home from the store, a baguette in my shoulder bag. I am supposed to be using this time to think of what I will write down about last summer, but the baguette has me thinking instead of the ham bone thawing and the pea soup we will make from it. Have I reminded Tony not to touch it, that it has to boil all afternoon for that soup? Yes I have, but did I leave a note as re-inforcement? I can picture him slicing the last scraps of meat from it for a ham sandwich, and my pace quickens. In that moment, I also see him tossing out the bone when he's finished.

Because he'd done that before, when we were still holding the big family dinners. After everyone had gone home, he stood in the kitchen, electric knife buzzing as he carved the remaining turkey meat from the bones — and then tossed the entire carcass into the garbage, forgetting we make stock from it. I had been horrified, a feeling that doubled when, apologizing, he began to root through the garbage to retrieve it.

I no sooner recall this than a second memory unfurls from the first, rippling further back through time along another path to another turkey dinner, this time in our old house, from before my mother went into care. This was a time when my father was taking on more of the meal preparations and Tony had promised him a large package of turkey meat for sandwiches. Instead, Dad got home to find he'd been given a bag of bones. I hate to think what went into the garbage that night.

The absent-minded professor, at it again.

The thought has stopped me in the middle of the sidewalk.

My sister and her husband would have been amused, just as they had been that time at my aunt's place when Tony momentarily mistook the sliding screen door for the older swinging style and pushed it hard, expecting it to slam shut behind him. Instead he stood blinking on the porch with the detached door clutched in both hands, to the roar of merriment around him. Was it around then, the 1990s, that my family started calling him the absent-minded professor?

Tony had always been a forgetful sort, and such missteps had worked their way into my subconscious, emerging in "Not Me," the short story that I mentioned earlier (see Appendix). It's about a woman and her sister, both afraid of inheriting Alzheimer's from their mother. As the plot twist, I gave it to the husband, instead.

I even gave him Tony's middle name, Josefus. It was published in a literary magazine in the summer of 1999, but it had taken a couple of years to write — I was teaching full-time then — and likely another year or two to send it around. So, perhaps 1995 was when the idea first struck, if not before. Tony would have been just forty-six years old.

This last series of memories has arrived like a landslide, flattening everything around it. So much for my plans to focus on how to write about last summer. I am so far off-course now, so much further back in time that, even though I slowly begin moving forward again, I linger in that distant past until I reach home, amazed at myself for having missed such obvious signs.

I find Tony sitting cross-legged on his office floor, eyes closed, meditating, the ham bone safe in the fridge. Once I plunge the bone into a pot of water and leave it on the stove to simmer, I call Tony to join me for lunch. Then I head to my desk and clear my thoughts to return to last summer. I don't need to make notes about the short story first. A copy of it has been sitting on the shelf above my desk all along, waiting for me to remember.

The days approaching the July long weekend of 2017 had been difficult. Tony had an earlier-than-usual deadline for the *Financial Post*, so he hurried to finish it, and sent copy that wasn't ready.

Racing to that deadline had been hard on him, upsetting his routine and his mood. He hit the desk as soon as he rose. He was abrupt, reclusive — well, he was behaving like many writers facing a deadline, with one exception: he was afraid.

Most writers can't stop talking about a project. They think everyone finds it as fascinating as they do. It haunts them. They tinker with it. They obsess. Tony, however, didn't talk about the project. I didn't know what it was about or who he had to interview. He complained loudly, but in vague terms about the lack of time, not about the content. He would burst out of his office to do so, only to return to it to waste time scrolling through the internet.

This was the same panic and avoidance he'd shown on those recent projects. Friends suggested I phone his editor and divulge his condition. One acquaintance even suggested I help him write the pieces. I knew I couldn't do that. Secretly, I wished the newspaper would just drop the column.

The editor promptly rejected the article, and I thought the moment had come. But no, she sent it back to him to rewrite, giving him one more day to do it. That would have been a snap for the old Tony, but now, one day wasn't nearly enough time.

Tony came undone. That's the best description I can think of.

For the next twenty-four hours or more, he hunched over his desk, he didn't shower, and he didn't go outside. He was fuming, breathing through his teeth, still ranting about time while he bolted back a quick meal at the kitchen bar. At last, he leapt up from that meal and said, that was it, he was done. He was going to tell her he couldn't do it.

It was only when he wrote about this experience a few days later, when he was still electric with the pain of it, that I realized all that had gone on. The writing is vivid, the agony tangible.

> Last week was awful. I tried to do what I always did, which was to hit a job — in this case, an article — with intensity, because the deadline had been moved up considerably and I didn't have time to let it percolate (she was going on vacation and they apparently weren't replacing her — instead it had to be in before she left — which must have put intense pressure on her.
>
> And I failed....miserably.

Essentially, I blew it. The interview was tough, because, for one, she was being very PR, which means everything was guarded and channeled, etc...the exact thing that makes for horrible storytelling. At the same time, I couldn't seem to focus: All I could think of was how I had to get this thing done quickly (I had wasted a day or two previously) and how hard it was to get it. The story definitely didn't write itself.

The premise was that she was operating a different kind of PR company, that ran alongside her main one — which concentrated on "brands" (i.e. fashion, etc) and other typical PR/marketing stuff. The different one concentrated on (to put it simply) "doing good." It worked with companies who were in the new giving field, which generally meant for profit or not for profit companies that were formed and operated to help solve social problems (such as illiteracy, housing, clean water, etc.), largely in the U.S but also worldwide.

It sounded good on paper, but it all came across as murky in reality. It seemed that either she wasn't explaining it well, or I was asking all the wrong questions (I really had no idea what she was doing — may have forgotten it, and she thought I did because she apparently had talked about it with me before). Anyway, I was in a hurry, in a fog, I guess, and came away with a bunch of notes that really didn't hang together as a story.

But because I was on a deadline — as I was writing it had to be in the next day, I smashed something together from what little notes I had, and even ripped a piece of explanation off their website. I sent it in hoping it would pass (I had assigned pictures for it).

The result, as you know, was horrible. She rejected it, taking it apart piece by piece — to my mortification because I have been an editor and it was clearly garbage. But she did give me a day to fix it and send it in.

So, result: I was under pressure, fought with it all day, was in high agitation (resulting in much complaining, arguing, and fighting with you), and all the time worrying what this would all mean.

Worse, I was aware that I couldn't do it as easily as I once could, maybe couldn't do it at all. And, even more worse, I was going to miss a deadline, which I had never done in 40-plus years. That, combined with my general anxiety about my writing convinced me that I was unable to do it.

I was failing. I was old. My condition had reached one of the ultimate milestones — that I would have to give up the last real job of my older life, and career. Of course that also meant a monetary loss, albeit not a severe one.

In a spectacular flameout, I was confronted with the reality. It was over. I had lost the battle.

And now, you were upset and hurting, I was seething (and hurting), and I had to face the truth.

So I contacted her (at your suggestion) and told here I couldn't do it, that there wasn't enough time, and why didn't we just skip it for this month and she could run it the next month.

Then, feeling very defeated and broken, I went back out and sat with you, oblivious to the fact that you were feeling pretty broken and hurt after my raging and the huge fight we had. I even went back at one point and tried to finish it. But I gave up.

What was done was done, and, when the frenzy of anger, sorrow, self-loathing, fear and rage had left me, I felt what can only be described as relief.

I had done it. Crossed the line from trying to continue as if nothing happened to acceptance that it could very well be over.

And now, to tell you the truth, a sense of peace has come over me. The rage, and the loss, was a kind of catharsis, a seeing of the light on the road to Damascus. A strong pointer to the future instead of a remnant of the past.

I am now okay with it all. If she complains or questions me I will simply give it up. If she suggests it, I I will work at it until the end of the year. If not, then immediately (after I finish this piece of course).

I am 68 years old, and while I know many people who continue to work in their seventies, I am realizing that I can't. At least not that kind of work.

I have had strong thoughts and inklings of this for some time, but always ignored them, insisting that I could still keep up, and this condition wasn't going to affect my life.

But I realize now that it does. That life is over.

And, I hope, a new one is beginning.

I never heard back from her

I was relieved as well. Much of the arguing and hurt feelings that Tony describes above had not occurred between us, at least not to my recollection, but, I suspect, there had been a battle raging inside his own head. I also hadn't suggested he tell his editor he couldn't do it, though I was certainly glad he had. For two full years after he had been prescribed Aricept, he had continued to write for the *Financial Post*, which is an indication not only of his inherent abilities but of just how hard he pushed himself. His whole body, not to mention his brain, must have been exhausted with the effort.

Now, calm settled over the household. As I had mentioned in the previous email exchange with Tony, the gods had been generous in giving us two out-of-town weddings to attend in August — the celebrations arrived at just the right time, injecting a joyful mood into our lives.

We flew to Toronto for the first wedding. Tony's nephew Jacob was marrying a lovely young woman named Michele. It was a large celebration in the Jewish tradition — food and more food and dancing. It was good to see his elder sister, Josée, mother of the groom, happy and proud. She had lost her husband, Jerry, just two years before, so her stepsons Andy and Dan, the same Dan we had visited in Barcelona, escorted her down the aisle.

Tony is still a social butterfly, and he had a good time. Several guests commented that he seemed just fine. I was learning to smile at such comments and even be grateful that he could enjoy himself as much as the rest of us did. This was especially so after that July. The fact that we were in the same city that produced the *Financial Post* didn't seem to strike Tony, and I wasn't about to remind him.

Cinda and Godwin drove us around while we were there — we were staying at their new place just outside Toronto — and they got to see him when he wasn't "on," his frequent declarations of "This is new. I've never seen this!" when we were driving the same route, one full of heritage buildings. At the wedding, Godwin had carefully redirected Tony when, ever enthusiastic, he knocked back the traditional Scotch given to the men, and reached for another.

Except for going through security and walking off without his suitcase, which resulted in a mad dash back before our plane left, the return home went well, though Tony was tired.


It was an eventful August. As noted in our June email exchange, the gerontologist had, with Lorraine's counsel, filled out another Disability Tax Credit application. That was several months after our January appointment, and now, at last, in late August, it was approved. This time, she had written: "Mr. Wanless has dementia so his disability is not reflected in ADLs, but he is unable to work and his wife has to supervise decision-making and all his instrumental activities of daily living."

Bingo.

It didn't specify Alzheimer's, one of many diseases that fall under the term *dementia*. It seems it didn't have to. The approval was retroactive to 2015, when she had first prescribed Aricept. Once again I recall her words that day: We know what this is for.

We finally did.


We had another appointment with the gerontologist about a week after we returned from the wedding, and I felt some guilt at having gone behind her back to see the neurologist in the spring. After all, it was her comments and signature that had eventually completed the tax credit paperwork successfully. However, I was also becoming combative when I saw obstacles to Tony's treatment, so I was prepared. I quickly thanked her for filling out the form and told her our application had been approved.

She noted that we had been to see the neurologist and questioned our need to see both the neurologist and her.

We needed the MRI, I said.

She said she would have ordered one.

I told her that we had asked, and she had said no.

She said that she would have, had we asked again.

Emboldened by this, I pressed once more for her to enact the power of attorney. Again she was reluctant to draw up such a letter, and turned to Tony.

I should add here that it is extremely awkward to have to ask these questions in front of Tony, who at the time still felt he was more or less fine. A technique I have mentioned before, and used, recommended to me by my neighbour Olga, involved writing a note expressing my concerns to the doctor beforehand, which she could refer to discreetly in the meeting. But by this point I was truly running on empty, and had not had time for that.

She asked Tony some basic financial questions. He was way off on the value of our apartment, what his income totalled, and what payments we made in a month. It was the last question, though, regarding the spending of money, that triggered an explosive reaction. He roared at her about prices and costs and all the money that had to be paid for household expenses.

Rather than feel intimidated by such anger, I was delighted. He was showing the doctor exactly what I was witnessing at home, alone, when he was under a full Alzheimer's rage.

Finally, the gerontologist said, Tony! We all have to pay, and none of us *likes* it.

Then she turned to me and said, I'll write you that letter.

That was the turning point for us and this doctor. I felt that she finally saw what was going on at home. She would later acknowledge that we were in crisis, but that Tony's intelligence had allowed him to pull the wool over doctors' eyes.

Her letter arrived soon after. It contained the phrase "diagnosis of probable dementia." I would have preferred more forceful phrasing; however, no bank has ever questioned the probability.

We rested up for the remainder of August and then set off to Victoria for the second wedding. Devon, son of our friends Mary Beth and Michael, was marrying Alanna, a young woman we would soon meet and quickly like. Our friends threw a great party the night before the wedding, in their penthouse suite facing the harbour. Several friends I had worked with at Total Ed, an alternative school, were there. After we all left the school, we used to hold get-togethers they called "Ladies Lunches." I've never liked the term, but I loved the lunches. Now, to accommodate my changed situation, these include the men. All of us spent the entire evening out on the large patio, watching the ships lit up like Christmas trees, and the sun setting over the ocean. The ceremony and reception the next day took place in an old church in the country. Again, Tony had a great time, and when we rode back to the hotel we helped carry up all the wedding gifts. Mary Beth invited us in for a nightcap and suggested we sit out on the patio, again, to which Tony said in surprise, You have a patio?

His comment fell like a thunderclap on all of us who had been on that patio for several hours the previous night. Mary Beth was about to tease him and then stopped, realizing that yes, he had forgotten all about it. Good friends that they are, everyone jumped right in and said how great a nightcap would be and the laughter and conversation got rolling again.

In an email to Cinda a few weeks later, Tony wrote about something I hadn't considered. It had been a long, hot summer with smoke from forest fires drifting down from the mountains into the city of Vancouver, all of which had a negative impact on his cognitive health.

He was also blunt about marital ups and downs.

Hi again:

Sorry for the last problem with my email. I've been having a lot of computer trouble lately: really slow, all my connections seem to be scrambled, something on there is holding up things, and of course, half my buttons don't work, and the turn-onturnoff button is almost gone. I've been trying to clear stuff out of it, but it's not enough.

I'm going to have to get it serviced somehow.

Anyway, it's been going okay: lazy days of summer and all that. I wish I could say that made it fun, but it didn't really..... it just made it lazy. It's been pretty hot this year, and the fires are still raging out in the woods as we speak (today is particularly smokey — everything is under or behind a gray haze. And it is really hot. But they say rain will come soon.

The trip to TO was such a great break and I got to see a lot of the city I haven't really been to for years. So much has changed since I lived there almost 40 years ago. (God, it's weird saying that.)

Went to another wedding on the weekend — in Victoria where the son of an old friend of June's, someone she worked with for years, was marrying a Victoria woman. Strange, in a sense, because I hadn't seen him for years. He's all grown up now, tall, muscled and good looking — works out in the woods a lot as some kind of scientist.

Nice to see a lot of the old gang, including Karl, the BCTV cameraman who I used to run with when I worked there.

Big, wild guy, and it didn't take us long to get into crazy stuff. Loosened everybody up, including me.

It was also nice to get a break from all this brain problem stuff that seems to be swirling around. Now that I apparently officially have Alzheimers, I seem to be on this endless regime of doctors or sitting in a corner doing nothing in case I screw up.

Also, I gave up the last job I had — the column with the National Post finance section — after a particularly difficult article I did that was rejected because, frankly, it was just a mess — a tough interview subject, and at the same time, I was off in a fog for most of the summer — which of course led to even more restrictions on my life.

In a way it was dispiriting because it seems I just sit around sucking my thumb unless I'm ordered to do something domestic such as carrying stuff for June, etc. We seem to be having trouble here in the transition: She seems to be angry at me often, while I get angry back for being treated like a dolt (which, frankly I am sometimes — I don't really listen much and my hearing is going). She's working to0 hard, shouldering too much of the load, and so gets pretty frazzled and testy, and I, of course don't help matters much by saying that she shouldn't do so much and to leave stuff for later. Clash of styles. I also point out that if she insists on doing everything, I will let her, and she shouldn't get angry that she has to do everything.

blah blah blah. You know how it goes. Heat, too much to do (ie commitments), etc.

It's been a bad summer here all around. Very hot, and my back has been hurting for much of it — pulled, tore or badly strained a muscle (or more) in my back or hip — plus have some arthritis in the knees —so one has to curtails one's movements (ie exercise) and as a result starts to wallow in lassitude.

Not good for the mood or the brain.

I went to a physiotherapist, and he noted the muscle in the one leg with the problem (the whole left side, was atrophied, so obviously I have been favoring it, which probably means I'm off kilter. So I now have exercises to build up the knee. Even knowing it can be done is a relief. It was starting to impact everything, including my thinking.

I'm doing some jobs with the local community centre, writing a monthly literacy column, and filling in for the ESL guy when he's away. But this summer it has been kind of confusing, and then I had to go away to the wedding and so missed a session (they found some tutor to fill in) and it's apparently becoming unwieldy. Also, I seem a bit more confused lately (did I say it was hot? And that I haven't had any exercise for many weeks?Endlessly swallowing pa of oxygen really makes one stupid). So that's not been working out great either. Mostly I just want to lay around.

But September's here now, and while the forest fire smoke turns the sun red every day and it looks cloudy all the time, they say rain is on the way and so might clear thing up. It's been a hard summer.

But I'm starting to look at my routines again, pick up where I have left off, clean up, sort and throw out useless stuff — I try to purge regularly but have neglected it for some time —. The simpler I can make life, the better. One way to do that is spend absolutely nothing that I don't "HAVE" to spend. That simplifies considerably.

Also, our continual efforts to get some kind of government disability continues with a few indications of success. I now have disability tax credit, I believe. But they're being bureaucratic about other stuff. Same provincially, only worse. F'ing Socreds — spent all their time cutting everybody off everything. We'll see if the NDP (who barely scraped in during the last election) can change much, but I'm not expecting it. They have too flimsy a margin, and far too many people (ie unions and hard rock supporters) grasping for their share of the spoils. But hope springs eternal.

So how are things going there? Anything exciting? Get around much? You guys seemed to like it there, settled in and all that and developed some routines. I hope the winter won't be too hard in changing this.

It was so nice to see you guys. Life has changed since you left.

Take care, say hello to Godwin, and the whole gang.

Tony

The summer weddings were the highlight of a year that had held some dark moments. I had hoped the reflected glow would spill over into the fall.

It didn't last.

Much to my shock — no, dismay is a better word — Tony accepted another assignment passed along to him through a former journalism colleague.

This time I did step in, arguing, pleading, discouraging him from taking it, reminding him how hard it had been on him the last time, and how his gerontologist had warned him not to place so much stress on his cognitive system ... but he was determined to try again, and so the pandemonium began yet again, with predictable results.

It was a dreadful thing to watch.

# WHEN A WRITER CAN
# NO LONGER WRITE

Picture a fight in a schoolyard or outside a bar, maybe something you've seen in a movie. One guy is getting pummelled but keeps getting back up. As much as you might admire his pluck, you might also be somewhat appalled at the spectacle. Because it's ugly, and you wish he would just stay the hell down and end it.

Tony wouldn't stay down. He tackled the new assignment as he had the past ones, full of confidence in the task. He shut himself away in his office, begrudging the occasions he had to go to Paul's Club, or any other place he usually enjoyed. It was the loss of potential writing hours, he said. He was too busy, he said. He didn't have enough time.

Cinda arrived in October to visit Tony and to give me a break. I went on a writing retreat at Historic Joy Kogawa House for several days, and then attended a few events at the Vancouver Writers Fest.

She said the whole time I was away Tony had been busy working on his article, but when I returned, I found that he had been struggling with it, and not letting on. In particular, he'd had communication problems with the person he was interviewing, a misunderstanding about the subject matter, and so he had to re-do it.

I was seeing a familiar pattern. Staying up late, hunched over his computer, no exercise, eating frantically, neglecting to shower, his office an explosion of clothing and papers and file folders.

The final blow arrived when the person he was interviewing contacted the editor and demanded the piece be re-assigned to another writer. Tony was devastated. He had done everything in his power to come back swinging from his "spectacular flameout," but nothing had worked. Eventually, he agreed that enough was enough. He had to stop accepting such assignments. Fortunately, none came along to tempt him.

A month later, I encouraged him to put his writing efforts into *Four Umbrellas*. Tony got busy, and in a few days, had a piece for me that he would send by email.

L, he wrote.

A few minutes later he sent a second note:

L

And then a third time,

L

A few days later he successfully sent an email to me:

I now admit I have alzheimer's. I have to — the evidence is getting too strong. I am becoming more forgetful, of more things, and more often. Commonly, someone like you at home, or someone else elsewhere, will tell me something and an hour or two later I'll forget it (an hour or two? I'm being generous. Heck sometimes it's 20 minutes).

I know and people tell me that it's not unusual for people to forget names or conversations, but mine is more than that. I forget many things. I go to groups I belong to, and I remember the names of only one or two people, and sometimes they fade a bit too. Again, people will say that so what, that's not uncommon. But I should know these names — I have been seeing these people every week for some time, so they are not passing acquaintances (There is a woman in my group, and we ride transit together every week after group.....and I never remember her name (in fact I can't think of it now). I can picture her well, know a lot about her and her life, but, for the life of me I can't remember her name, even though I have, several times, sneakily looked it up or asked someone.

That's the kind of thing that, when coupled with other inci-dents of confusion — getting lost or "zoning out", while on the bus going to some familiar place (i.e.where my group meets) , for example, or leaving Paul's club for Yaletown and not realizing it was around the corner, so I ended up walking all over the place around it before I found it. Sure it had been a while since I went there, but I should have recognized that our group often ends up at a gelato place after a walk, and it's in Yaletown, albeit on the edge in a place I usually don't think of because it's not on the main drag. I noticed recently and thought "wow, I didn't know that" maybe I should have looked more carefully.

Actually, I find that happens a lot — my not noticing things, I mean. Places I've been to and where they are;

how I get there or to other familiar places that now aren't
so familiar, etc. It seems that I am inside my own head all
the time — not thinking or much else — but just focusing
on what is closely around me — and so no longer have
those mental maps that we all have. That sure sounds
like Alzheimers to me

Well, Tony was not about to give up entirely. He was writing
for a neighbourhood newsletter, the one he had mentioned in
the email to Cinda, a monthly piece aimed at English learners.
The subject matter has to be simple, the language uncomplicat-
ed. Perfect.

Renfrew Ravine
By Tony Wanless

Residents of Renfrew-Collingwood can consider themselves lucky because in their neighbourhood is an oasis
of nature and calm that acts as a relief from the usual
city noise and energy

    The Renfrew Ravine is an urban jewel — a little bit
of wilderness that is a reminder of what all of Vancouver
once looked like.

    This section of forest and stream sits surrounded by
busy streets with car, truck and transit noise and all the
other sounds that are a feature of daily life in a city.

    It reminds us that, not long ago, Vancouver was a
lush wilderness teeming with birds, animals and fish,
and which was home to many Native peoples....

He continues to write the column, though meeting deadlines is
on ongoing problem because they slip from his mind. As well, he

still volunteers a few times a year to fill in as leader of an ESL class at the same neighbourhood house.

It brings its own complications.

More than once he has had a student pop into his tai chi session next door to tell him he had forgotten the ESL class and that everyone had left.

On one occasion, he filled in for the regular guy, as arranged, but then wanted to leave our place after dark to return the binder of materials so the instructor would have them in the morning.

I said that was not a good idea, and that he should wait until morning as he was heading there for tai chi classes, anyway. He felt constricted and I heard more of the thumb-sucking comments that had appeared in that email to his sister. He stormed off to his office but returned an hour or so later, calmed, and said brightly that there was no problem, after all. He had already handed in the binder of papers.

I forgot, he said.

Well, what could we do in that moment but laugh?

This aspect of the disease has its upside. I have learned that if I let a discussion stop before it builds into a full-blown argument, and just wait, he soon forgets all about it.

That doesn't mean we don't still argue. I know that a caregiver is never supposed to argue with a person with Alzheimer's, regardless of the subject. Things will only escalate because the ability to reason, to be logical, is not always present in that person. But along with memory loss and visuospatial issues comes paranoia, and I find it difficult to hear accusations and not defend myself:

No, I have not taken your medication and hidden it.

No, I haven't left the broken door as punishment for you breaking it. We need to hire someone to install a new one.

Sometimes my explanations make perfect sense to him, and sometimes they lead to an escalation of feelings. In the case of the pills, when I managed to locate where he had stashed them, in a corner of the bottom floor of the pantry, he saw my finding them as proof that I'd hidden them.

And I'm human. Sometimes I become exasperated, even angry. Why would I hide his pills? Here, I wanted to say. Take ten of them!

We had a heated discussion the other day when Tony broke a glass. Everyone has watched a plate or glass slip from their hands. Accidents happen. But breakage happens frequently around here. A person with visuospatial problems can't be expected to wash or dry fragile items, so I ask Tony to leave them for me and focus on the pots and pans, instead.

And what is the matter with me that I think he will remember?

He only remembers the instant the glass snaps in his hands, and in his defence he goes on the attack. It's just cheap glass, he says, what do you care? I say it could cost two bucks or two hundred, the point is I keep asking you not to wash the delicate stuff, I'll do it. Why do we even have it? he counters. We should just get rid of it.

And around and around we go.

Of course, the simple solution is to pack it all away, but when that happens it means I will have given up, and that will be a hard moment to bear. Because it's not just the glass that's in pieces, is it?


When we walked along that beach discussing the idea of this book, Tony was convinced that all he had was a fixable condition called MCI, and only after several months of appointments and tests, along with the sheer evidence of gaps and cognitive glitches that marked our lives, was he able to accept the probable cause: Alzheimer's. From the very start, I had envisioned us writing back and forth to each other, just as I also wondered if that was even possible. A few pages in, I knew it wasn't, and I had to shift my approach, not showing him the narrative in progress, so that his recollection of events could be written independently of mine. Over time, as Tony's condition worsened, I had to consider not only that he could not take part in structuring the narrative or editing the results, but also that the organizational details that were confounding him in his freelance writing, leading to his "spectacular flameout," were the very skills required of this project.

We needed to sort this out, not only in conversation, which we had attempted several times, with each time forgotten by him, but now in writing, where we could both refer to what the other had said. And so began another email exchange:

February 16, 2018

We have been working on this for almost a year. I can see us continuing with same for another year, an easy exchange of comments back and forth. I would hate for us to record all these thoughts and do nothing with them. Should we reach a point where the organization of the material is overwhelming for you, or you lose interest, I would like to continue working on the project, in areas of both writing and editing. Okay?

For now, please don't worry about writing anything else. Just tackle the above question, and then we're off to the races.

February 18, 2018

First: I am astonished that it has been a year.....and am also somewhat ashamed because I feel like I have let the side down, am a failure, blew it, etc., because I never really allowed myself to be in it with any depth. I treated it more like a diary of the day, than a real exploration of the situation.

Okay, maybe that is being a bit harsh, but I do believe I really wasn't approaching it the way I should have. Whether that is because I was afraid to, didn't know how to, or was simply too lazy to, I don't know. I do know that I seemed to mostly be stuck on the "I really want to do something here" and never really figured out what that was, so just did a reporting job. Maybe, after all these years, that's all I have become. Anyway, I am going to try from now on to add a little depth and try to stick to the topic at hand.

As to your question: Yes, of course, continue if I can't, or don't want to. I don't think the latter will happen, however. In fact, I am hoping for the opposite.

I suspect there have been problems because I am not sure what I was supposed to be writing: was it heart-and-soul feelings about "my condition" and, my current state in life, or what?; was it merely creating diary entries, most times (but not always) with some relation to your question; was it some feeble attempt to co-ordinate various streams of thought? Was it a mish-mash of all three.

Simply, I think I never, as the vernacular had it, "was into it". Also, I am not sure how to write any more, at least not with purpose. I think, after a lifetime or being "around" the arts, I may have calcified into a mere talker, a gabbler, a smartmouth with little substance.

But I would like to re-learn, to go back to that state where words and their use in delineating feelings and thoughts are important and then should become (almost) art. I fear too often that I was in journalism too long, forgot how to write with emotion, and, simply, lost it.

(Maybe I never had it — I was simply good at distantly and occasionally wringing emotion and "soul"out of others' situations, but not out of my own. Or perhaps it was that I was good at writing with a superficially that only little depth.)

I do want to make this into something worthwhile. I long to be a good "diarist" who can make myself and readers understand our emotions, thoughts, fears, etc that flow now, when I am at the nadir of my life. And I fear that I ... I cannot any more, or that I was ever really able to.

Might I suggest that we sit down and work out what you are looking for, and what I perceive, etc.?

February 19, 2018

Yes in almost three weeks it will be a year. As you suggested, we sat down last night with cups of coffee and pencils and paper and discussed what I am looking for in this project, and what you perceive to be its purpose.

I began the chat by quoting the Maurice Chevalier and Sophie Tucker duet "I Remember it Well," with each line offering vastly differing recollections of past moments, always ending with the titular line.

Not! you added. And we laughed. Because, where two people will always have different recollections of any given event, our situation has the added dimension that your memory is compromised by cognitive difficulties, or, as you put it, "I can't remember anything. I can't remember anyone's names!"

So, what are we trying to do with this project? Last night I said again that this is a way for you to tell readers what it's like to have Alzheimer's. It's a unique opportunity to describe it not just from the caretaker's point of view (mine) but also from the viewpoint of the person with the disease (you). And as I've said, some readers might be surprised at how capable you still are, that you can take part in a writing project such as this. And again, it's your disease, but it's a shared experience, our journey.

We laughed again when we saw ourselves enacting our roles in this project: I, hunched forward, clipboard on my knees, scribbling down my ideas and yours; you, notebook quickly abandoned, leaning back against the cushions like a philosopher, arms waving as you talked. And then you admitted that you were nervous, worried that you couldn't make writing decisions anymore and that you wrote everything in a hurry without reading it over before sending. I said being in a hurry is a good metaphor for what you must be feeling, wanting to get everything out and on the page while you still can. And you said yes, exactly. And on that note, thank you for answering my question, that yes, it's okay for me to continue if you can't or won't, though you doubt it will be the latter.

So, here is what you said you want with this project. "I want to do something," you said last night, "do talks about this." We agreed that this book would be an obvious vehicle, the means for getting out in public to discuss and answer questions about your experience with Alzheimer's. For instance, you said you'd like to, "Tell what it's like when you see signs in yourself. I can tell you right now that it never occurs to anyone that they might have Alzheimer's." You

could offer not only detailed descriptions of what this journey has been like for you, but also offer tips, tell everyone
what has helped you.

You said a good place to begin would be the pills incident.
I've told what it was like from my perspective: confusing
and a little frightening to be accused of taking the very
things that help you and that I want you to take. But you
said it had more to do with loss of control and the panic
that ensued. Over to you.

February 10, 2018 [March 2018]

Much to talk about here. But first let me apologize, because I messed up somehow on this computer and the
thread became all mixed up, with 2017 apparently being
on top, and this in 2018 a few posts later. I get confused
whenever I try to respond, because I can't determine what
I am responding to. I'm not even sure when I started this
post, although I think it was near the beginning of the
year. And now it's just turned to March.

Because I get so frustrated by this, and can't seem to get
into various parts for some reason, I'm going to have to
ask you to re-order it. At one time this would have been
easy, but now I am bewildered by the Microsoft system.

Anyway, I hope that, in some way, I can explain why the
long delay.

The simple answer was that it the end of the year and
the start of a new one (2017—isn't that the future, how

did that happen), which meant many other things to think about and do.

The not-so-simple answer is much more complicated and might describe some of what's going on.

The end of the year was the time I realized where I was in life. I know that sounds grand and pompous, and it probably is to an extent. But I did realize something about myself over the past few months. I'm not sure if I can articulate that very well at this point, but I'll give it a try later. (and, since I wrote these past few paragraphs some time ago, I don't really remember what I was going to say.

I do apologize, but I'll try to pick up the thread.

First let me explain something about the new year, which might help you make some sense of it all. I was in my "I'm going to be a better person" phase, which commonly happens when the year turns — the difference this year was that it extended a bit longer then usual. This year, my "betterment" included plans to (re)learn French, change my approach to exercise, gain more control over my mind which involves more meditation. Then it was also to keep a running diary and thought calendar, separate from this one, change some bad habits, etc. etc. . Oh yeah, I wanted to enjoy life more!

Then, since I was sick of "plunging" and then becoming totally lost and quitting, I spent time planning all this stuff.

Now, excuses and mea culpas over, and I hope not to familiar and annoying, let's get at it.

So now it's march 7 and I'm barely back at it. By the way, I have already prioritized some of my plans, which means

I put a few so far down they might as well not exist. Sometimes experience does help.....I hope.

But, this is becoming a schoolboy's whine, so let's just pick it up now.

Turning to the task at hand I should answer your questions, each of which was a point of departure for a conversation, but none of which was carried continued or expanded. I think it was around the following point:

You said: "at a certain point I might have to take over this project.How do you feel about that? You have mentioned before your concerns about loss of control over decisions affecting your life. I also added that it might seem to the outside world that I am doing all this for my personal gain. Any comments?"

I guess the first thing I can say is ... well we were using different typefaces for some reason — again one of those computer things that I could have fixed in a jiffy at one time and now just makes me tired and grumpy just thinking about it.

Anyway, you asked how I would feel if you had to take over this project if I couldn't handle it any more (maybe apropos, considering my previous paragraph and request).

Hmm, I'm not sure if I feel anything about it. I think there was a time when I might have been angry and upset, because it was "another example of my loss of control over myself" (which, in hindsight, was a pretty stupid thought, but what can I say....my brain is scrambled, or so they tell me. I'm agreeing with them more often than I used to.)

But to get back to the point. I am fine with it now. I have become more stoic, more accepting, and less affected by change now than I was. Why this is, I'm not sure. I'm certain that acceptance of my state is one reason, and sheer fatigue caused by arguing over things that are either unimportant or inevitable is probably another. If you deem it to be best, then I'll go with it. But I don't really think I'm there yet. In fact I want to get back at this. I had a big of a plunge in spirit and energy there for a while (it was November and December!), but I believe I have conquered that but changing my life somewhat.

For example, I now instantly change typing and spelling mistakes, instead of just ignoring them(or not even noticing them, which is really really scary).

I also don't worry about many other things. I suppose it's about time that I reached this state of equanimity: After all I am going to be 69 years old in two weeks and that's supposed to come with the territory. It was exciting I guess when I was young to fight everything (and almost everybody) that seemed to impinge on my freedom, but now I have (I hope) learned that none of that really matters. What seemed like slights, insults, etc. in my youth that demanded a ferocious response to protect my self-sense) now seems silly and overly prideful.

Pride (at least not too much) is important when you are young and trying to establish yourself in life, your work, relationships, because you're not to certain about your qualities and abilities. But when you reach my — ahem — advanced age, you realize that's all silly. You don't have to convince people who you are. They already know that, even though it might not exactly align with your view. But then, who cares. It is, as they said in the old days, no matter. What they think is their purview, and what I think is mine.

Although, frankly, I don't think much about myself anymore. I know, I was pretty self-centered and prideful for years — a result of trying to convert myself from lowlife schmuck to venerable sagacity. (Hey we all need a self image. I prefer that one).

So, to get back to the point, all this prattle is really just a way of saying, if we get to the point where you think I can't do this any more I am willing to at least listen. I will still need to be convinced however, and that might involve some .... um ... vigorous debate. But in the end, if the proposition is adequately explained, I'll probably go along with it.

I'm not a fighter any more. It was good for the ego (and the hormones) in the old days, but I don't think there is need to put up the dukes for much today. I have become very philosophical, generally adopting much of the stoic mindset, and so see everything as just another phase of life, not to be taken as insult. From what I've seen, I gather it's common for older men to think "this too shall pass" about most things and so let them pass.

Is this just an older man ruminating about life, or is it a real line of thinking? I don't know. But it is a lot more peaceful than being angry all the time. Who knows, maybe if I am this way all the time, I may have a few years more than I think. I do know it is a nice way to be.

# PART FOUR

## DATELINE DIAGNOSIS

# BACK TO THE BEGINNING

We are just six weeks away from that blustery spring day when we will receive the final diagnosis that began the introduction and set this narrative in motion.

Just before that last email exchange, Tony and I had attended the day-long session of the neuropsychological memory tests, administered by one of the residents at the Centre for Brain Health. It really did take all day, with a short break for lunch, and Tony noted:

> That all-day testing at UBC hospital that we undertook last week was quite revealing — in some ways very different from what I had expects (although to be honest I didn't know what to expect.) For one, I didn't realize how tiring and taxing it would be. In the morning, I cruised through many of them, not being perfect but generally getting everything in the top percentile — I believe—.

There were a couple in which I was completely flummoxed (what a marvelous word!) however. These mostly had to do with very short-term memory, which I admit, has been facing considerably in recent months. But the afternoon tests were far less successful. I was very tired and as a result, very dulled, so put on a pretty anemic performance. The tester, a young guy just out of school but knowledgeably, interesting and eager, said this was often the case and I shouldn't be upset by it. Happens to everybody, etc.

I really wanted to believe him.

We have another couple of weeks of anticipation before we get the results from the same resident. We've already been told we won't see the neurologist until after that, when we will get a diagnosis based on the combined results of those day-long tests and the MRI that was taken back in August.

More hurry up and wait.

In the meantime, we have another appointment with the gerontologist.

When I tell her we won't get the MRI results until April, she says, Just a minute. She was sent a copy, and calls it up on her screen, where it hovers in black and white, that familiar butterfly shape within the slice of brain.

She points to the image and we look while she describes signs of mini-strokes and shrinkage in the temporal lobe area.

The evidence of strokes somewhat surprises me, if only because I have suspected them all along but never had confirmation. I didn't see my mother's MRI but was told by her doctor about the presence of mini-strokes. She had had a fall, too. So I ask this doctor if Tony's fall in 2011 was caused by one of these strokes, but apparently an MRI can't show that.

The doctor adds that the shrinkage, or atrophy, in the temporal lobe region is the hallmark of Alzheimer's disease.

Naturally, by this point, Tony and I are not surprised by that. He would later write:

> For a long time I resisted any offers, or even mentions, of help for my "condition" as we (I) secretly called it — Late. I have tried other names like Bob, etc., but have just settled on "Al." It's less work).
>
> Wasn't up to calling it by it's name — Alzheimer's— just yet. Even the fact that it was "Early" didn't get me to name it regularly. I mean, one doesn't go around saying "Hi, I'm Tony, I have Alzheimer's while secretly thinking "Booga Booga, (look out it might be catching!). Because that's the expression that many people try to hide, but are often unsuccessful when you confess that you might have it.
>
> But I'm past that now (he says, sounding very post "feeling" trained). You can call me a better person now. Of course I'm not , I've just been humbled.
>
> I mean it's very difficult concealing a problem when you constantly have to ask people their names even though they have told you several times, or have to ask what happened 10 minutes ago ("I wasn't really paying attention; I have a hearing problem in this ear; or the more blatant "who cares?"?
>
> But when you get down to it, I have become liberated from the shame monster. I have what I have, I am who I am, and there's not much I can do about it. And it works. I rarely see the horror cloud that I expected would come into people's eyes when I tell them. Maybe that cloud was more in my mind than theirs'.

This isn't unique to me of course. I believe that most people form a persona that they like and present to the world outside there own head. Sometimes they even grow to believe it really is them. That bully who is really a weakling inside; The "successful" person who is still trying to cover up a history of weirdness and wimpy-ness and rejection; the brave person, who's trying to compensate for fear, the "rich" person who's covering a childhood of aching poverty.

I also believe (hope) that there comes a time in everyone's life, when they can finally shed that cloak they're hiding behind and come out as the person they really are.

Now, I know that admitting you have a disease, even a sometimes-frightening one, is hardly up there with coming-out sexually, or some other incredibly wrenching life change. But it has its scary decision-making moments as well. Will they avoid me because they fear it might be catching; will they be overly helpful and start talking to me louder as if I was losing my hearing or something similar (ie, treating one as some kind of invalid); or aggressively helping me when I don't need i,t perhaps out of mistaking kindness, or more often to look like a good sport?

But it doesn't mean it's the end of your life. Actually, it's the beginning of a new one.

It took me a while to discover this, but it's been humbling. I always thought I was a somewhat hot shot, smart and quick, able to leap tall buildings with a single bound (sorry, I always loved that description of Superman from the old TV series.)

Having a life changeing condition, and that's what AI is, just makes you different than you were before. Much like age does. When you turned 30, were you the same as when you were a lusty, but not very aware 15-year-old? Of course not.

So now you are an — ahem — older man who might have a physical or mental problem that changes your life. So ride with the changes. Accept the fact that you are ridiculously annoying at times with your constant forgetfulness and your resulting endless questioning of your poor spouse or colleagues. Or that some of what you thought were your best traits have withered.

Because with that comes a different you: A little shop-worn, much slower, not as bright or capable in some areas, perhaps, but also calmer, more accepting, more humble, and, hopefully, kinder.

As they say, momento mori, shit happens, time changes everything, you can't beat it.

In the time you have left, why fight it. Life is a lot easier that way.

He has accepted the outcome. I'd anticipated it for years. What more was needed? And yet, since we have come this far we decide we might as well hear what the day-long tests show. For the same reason, we want to meet the neurologist next to learn if the combined results reveal anything further.

Once again, I am appalled by things that members of the medical profession will say. For one thing, when Tony says he has trouble remembering passwords the resident assures him that he does, too! I didn't find this at all helpful.

Yes, everyone from time to time forgets a password or loses a card, just as they might lose keys or a wallet, but for Tony this is a constant.

The resident then discusses the results, including that it seemed at times Tony showed a lack of focus, or effort.

I nod. Lack of focus is a well-recognized problem with any sort of cognitive issue.

He sums up the results by saying that, in his opinion, the test scores show more of a vascular issue than anything else.

You mean, from a stroke? I ask.

Yes, he says.

Tony is looking around the room so I lean forward and say that the gerontologist had looked at the MRI with us and pointed out the signs of atrophy, which indicate Alzheimer's.

He glances over a printed image of the MRI and confesses to not being an expert, but repeats that to him the signs indicate a vascular issue. That would be better, he says, than Alzheimer's.

As he walks us out, he talks about ways that parts of the brain can be re-routed. I think my mouth had fallen open for the entire way. I suspect that when we meet the neurologist in two months he will confirm what the gerontologist told us, and that the last thing we need to hear now is that another outcome will be better. How will that make us feel anything but worse? It's not like we can change the outcome with wishful thinking.

We won't see the resident again, as he is finishing up his term at the brain centre and heading elsewhere for further training. However, perhaps when Tony had been looking around the room he had been listening to the young man all along. A few days later, Tony astonishes me with a completely different version of that day from mine, writing that he is doing fine:

As we both noted in my lest checkup, I'm actually doing quite well. The MRI showed I had some problems in the front of my brain, which affected memory, but, for the most part, I'm doing fine. In fact, I'm still thinking that, with enough work, I can turn some that around, repair the damage, so to speak. I keep reading that with all the new neuroplasticity thinking that the brain can be regenerated. but it's a long hard slog and I'm not sure if it works on what I have. But one can only try, and besides it makes for a great life purpose, wouldn't your think. I mean it's far more purposeful than the long slow fade everyone else seems to think is in the cards.

It's April, and we are back to where this story started, heading out to the Djavad Mowafaghian Centre for Brain Health at UBC Hospital for the final, definitive diagnosis that we had been receiving in pieces over these years. In that respect, it will be a confirmation, not a revelation — at least for me.

It is also a full-circle moment in my own life. This is exactly where I had taken my mother, years before the construction of the beautiful centre with its soaring panes of glass etched with strings of brain cells like the tentacles of an octopus. The humbler hospital building is still there, beside the new one, and I would park right out front if there was room and if not, would drop my mother off at the curb because my father was there to take her inside to wait for me while I found parking.

Tony and I took the car once, parking in a large parkade within walking distance, but we found in the long run that the bus took not much longer, was cheaper, and convenient. The bus route didn't exist back when I took my mother there. On this day, Tony and I catch the bus just across the street from our apartment, and it passes our old house before winding its way west to drop us off right in front of the Centre for Brain Health.

Tony's diagnosis of dementia was retroactive to 2015, but three years later we are looking at specifics, at getting a diagnosis more firm than probable Alzheimer's.

As I mentioned earlier, *dementia* is an umbrella term covering a number of conditions, Alzheimer's being one of them. There is also frontolobal dementia, Lewy body dementia, vascular dementia, as well as mixed dementia, which has characteristics of Alzheimer's and vascular dementia. The Alzheimer Society of Canada also lists mild cognitive impairment, as well as diseases that can lead to dementia including Huntington's, Parkinson's, and multiple sclerosis.

Further, the Society discusses the reversibility of some dementias:

> A small percentage of dementias are reversible, occurring as a secondary development in treatable conditions. Toxic reactions to prescription or over the counter medications are the most common cause of reversible dementia. Others include dietary or vitamin B12 deficiencies, infections, tumours, alcoholism, inflammatory states, hormonal dysfunction, environmental toxins, drug abuse, and depression.

Tony had once clung to the idea that there was a possibility that the symptoms could be reversed. That he could beat this thing. This was before he was forced to accept that he had Alzheimer's, which is a dementia that is not reversible.

One month has passed since Tony wrote that he was doing fine, since the resident told us to hope for a diagnosis of vascular issues, as that would be a better outcome.

On this day in April, however, we receive the news that a better outcome no longer exists as a possibility; instead, we are told that we must accept the worse one. While it is expected, the very fact of it, confirmed by the day-long tests and the brief test and the MRI, truly cause me to stagger. I am unbalanced by the truth, thrown into the dizzying prospect of a future that is all too familiar to me.

In that moment, I feel cursed by the gods.

Again, I ask if the mini-strokes might have caused that fall in the kitchen, but the neurologist says the tests cannot determine that. He goes on to say that Alzheimer's is progressive and that life expectancy is seven to ten years from diagnosis. I pity him his job. No wonder doctors prolong giving the diagnosis.

Here, in part, is the written assessment we receive the following week:

> Mr. Wanless's cognitive symptoms continue to progress with time and are now significantly affecting his daily functioning. We think that his progressive symptoms, impaired daily functioning, declined cognitive testing scores, neuropsychological profile, and brain images are suggestive of an ongoing neurodegenerative disease of the Alzheimer's type.

As predictable as that analysis is, the report does contain one small surprise:

> Neuropsychological testing showed a normal intellect and average performance in most of the cognitive domains except for the memory where he performed poorly in both visual and verbal areas.

*Normal* and *average* are two words I would never have used to describe the bright mind of my husband, Tony Wanless. Alzheimer's has dulled his cognitive agility, doused the spark that once would have set his brain on fire at the very challenge of these tests. The doctors, however, never knew the old Tony, so they are seeing loss of memory as the key concern. Certainly, memory loss, on its own, is concern enough, but they are seeing the test results, not the man.

The SPECT scan, by the way, was reported to be normal, as was the CT scan.

# WHAT NEXT?

don't know how to write this. If this really is my story, too, then I should say more — not just about my role in writing this book but about my role, current and upcoming, in our shared life. I'd rather not. It's a role I take on reluctantly. I don't want to be a caregiver, not for the third time, and especially not for the man who has been my closest friend, my confidant, and was supposed to be my partner for the rest of my life. I don't want to think about this new future. I have enjoyed the process of going back, the leisurely pace of stopping to examine and muse. But going forward requires courage, and I'm a coward. I will spend the remaining years of my life alone. Money will be tight. I have a sense of what that will be like because the process began years ago, and I'm afraid. I'd crawl under the bed and hide if the snakes hadn't beat me to it. I miss him already and maybe I shouldn't write that, either, because he will read it, and then forget he read it, which is even worse.

The year 2017 had been a low one for me. I scrawled in a notebook that I simply couldn't handle any more. On top of this, my 2017 had been very much like Tony's 2008. My writing was going nowhere and my teaching jobs had dried up. As it turned out, this was not altogether a bad thing. Our days were filled with one medical appointment after another. Tony could no longer go to these appointments unaccompanied. He couldn't remember the dates and times any more than he could find the locations, which underscores the irony that we were still without a firm diagnosis then. Also, his worsening condition compelled me to put fiction aside to focus on the more time-sensitive book: this one.

I wouldn't have been able to do much else in the way of work during this time; however, I could have done some. It would have been a welcome and healthy break.

With the final diagnosis in 2018, the appointments settle down to a manageable level, and a break does come my way. Shortly after our visit to UBC, I come upon a job listing. It seems ideal for me, given my background in both writing and working with an at-risk population. I apply, and get the job facilitating writing workshops at a treatment centre for addiction. It's part-time, close to our home, and supplies a badly needed cash injection.

A shift occurred, I wrote in that notebook, a very subtle one, but finally, I could breathe.

What I have achieved is balance.

I didn't get to that point alone.

For one thing, the neurologist noted matter-of-factly that I would need help, and set me up with a social worker, who in turn arranged a case manager for us. She came over to our apartment and gave Tony a simple three-word memory test, such as man, car, hat, and he scored zero.

She approved us for home support. This was to relieve me when I needed to go out to meetings and other functions. When the social worker heard that this was my third time being a care-giver for someone with dementia, she also sent me to a psychi-atrist for counselling, who enrolled me in a mindfulness course aimed at relieving stress in caregivers. All of the above filled a calendar year; none of it would have happened without the MRI and diagnosis.

All along, the eldest of my sisters-in-law, Josée, who regularly donates to Paul's Club's baseball fundraiser each summer, has been providing additional financial support for Tony, while the young-est, Cinda, flies out once or twice a year to provide me with a badly needed respite.

For another thing, Tony started attending more days at Paul's Club, and the organizers, Nita and Michael, have arranged for him to arrive at the same time on Tuesday as program director Chelsea, so that I can get to work on time. Without them, I couldn't have accepted the job. Without a recommendation from Mary Beth, who counselled some of the at-risk youths I taught, I wouldn't have been offered the job. Without the understanding of Dale, who interviewed me and then waited to hear if I could make ar-rangements for Tony, the job would have gone to someone else.

Finally, without the help of Garth and Joni, and of Terri, how could I have worked over Christmas? Paul's Club closes for the hol-idays, but the treatment centre, of course, never does. They came over to hang out with Tony so I could go to work.

My job has lifted my spirits, and, in so doing, has probably made me a better caregiver. It inspires me to see the courage and conviction it takes for the clients, my students, to recover from addiction, and to know that while drug and alcohol abuse damages the brain, it is one of the few instances where improvement of cognitive function is possible, as long as they stay clean and sober. There is hope for them. That is a gift that they are likely unaware they are holding, and it's one I wish I could give to Tony.

This reminds me that the doctors at the brain centre are concerned about Tony's depression and his test answers that suggested suicidal ideation but no intent. In his last appointment, they asked Tony face-to-face if he ever thought about suicide. Tony shrugged and said something like, Doesn't everyone at some point?

Exactly, I thought.

I was sitting right there and I waited for them to ask me, but they didn't. No doctor ever has, not even my own, but I suspect that many caregivers have contemplated a number of solutions for the grief and stress they are feeling, and hovered over that one, even briefly. Why don't doctors ask?

They should, because there is a cost to caregiving. Recently, I found a pamphlet from the Alzheimer Society of Canada on reducing caregiver stress. It involves ten warning signs:

1. Denial
2. Anger
3. Withdrawing socially
4. Anxiety
5. Depression
6. Exhaustion
7. Sleeplessness
8. Emotional reactions
9. Lack of concentration
10. Health problems

It is remarkably similar to the stages of grief, although, equally remarkable, grief is not listed. At our support group meetings, though, we discuss what is called "silent grief."

It is the same term I used to describe how secretive Tony and I were about his disease.

We use the term in the support group to describe our feelings. Your partner, while still alive, is not the same person any more, and the relationship has had to shift to accommodate this. You function as any widow or widower would: all tasks and decisions, financial and otherwise, are made by you alone, and yet you must also gather up every last drop of patience to deal with the person very much present with his repeated questions or her looping of behaviour, and the lost items, the damaged or broken equipment, plugged plumbing, repair bills.

Also, the person in your care might think he doesn't need it; she might think you are the one with the problem.

There is a financial cost to caregiving. The Provincial Guide to Dementia Care in British Columbia states: "In 2011, caregivers in Canada provided over four hundred million unpaid hours looking after someone with dementia." These statistics come from the Alzheimer Society of Canada study, "A New Way of Looking at the Impact of Dementia in Canada," published in September 2012.

Of these caregivers, the majority were women. An April 13, 2019 article in the *Globe and Mail* reported the findings of a Statistics Canada study in which it is stated that the proportion of women caregivers was three times that of men in 2015.

Reduced work hours during child-bearing years already compromise a woman's income and pensionable earnings. Caregiving further erodes a woman's financial security. I am a typical example. I stayed home with my son for the first few years of his life before returning to work, then I went part-time, and then I took leave to both write and help care for my mother, then for my father, and now I work part-time while I care for my husband.

There are other costs. Depression, isolation, grief, all take their toll on the cognitive system.

There is also a frightening fact: those who care for people with Alzheimer's stand a greater risk of developing the disease than others their age who are not caregivers — they are six times more likely, according to a study out of Utah and reported by the *Journal of the American Geriatric Society* in 2010.

I am no saint, despite the praise heaped on me for my patience by my sisters-in-law, Josée and Cinda. I reach my breaking point as anyone else would. I go for short walks when the conflict becomes too much, and, much as when I let a few minutes elapse following a heated discussion, I can then return to a new, calm Tony. I try to practise mindfulness and meditation to calm myself. I have also tried to dodge conflict, sometimes to laughable effect.

Tony has taken to tearing open new packages of toilet paper and stacking them unsteadily on the wicker shelf above the toilet. I call it Toilet Paper Mountain, and watch with a shudder as the inevitable tremor sends toilet paper tumbling down and rolling all over the floor. We discuss this to no effect. I buy more toilet paper; he insists on tearing the package open and building Toilet Paper Mountain once again. To circumvent this, I hide the next new package in an upper cupboard. Problem? We have high ceilings. If I ask for Tony's help, he'll know what I'm doing and then build another damn mountain. So, to avoid drawing his attention, I grab a little stool from the bedroom and stand on it. Not quite tall enough, I stand on my tiptoes and stretch … and the stool slides out from under me and I fall onto its upended legs, hitting my chin, elbow, and shin. The bruises are ugly, but when I start describing the problem to my support group I hear its ridiculousness, that I would injure myself so badly over something called Toilet Paper Mountain, and we all have a laugh. My lesson? Think it through, first. And for God's sake, find a lower shelf, which I've done, in a location that shall remain undisclosed as Tony will be reading this.

When people hear that my husband has Alzheimer's, they often tell me about a parent or grandparent who has it. I know from personal experience how hard that can be, but it's not the same.

With grandparents and even parents, you might put in a full day driving them to appointments and picking up a prescription as well as groceries along the way, setting up a time for a support worker to stop in that night. And then you go home, and if you're lucky, your spouse greets you in the kitchen with a glass of wine and puts a steak on the grill, and for a few short hours, until that dreaded midnight call, you are home, safe — you can relax.

There is no safe place when it's your spouse with dementia. Home becomes the battleground. Strife, disagreement, and even the potential for violence are lurking. The younger he or she is, the more physical power behind the violence. There are ways to avoid some of that. Never argue with someone with Alzheimer's, as I've noted. Change the subject, even offer a cup of tea, and like a zap from the heavens the mood can swiftly change.

Even so, when it's your spouse, you bring the caregiving home in ways that those with parents living in the same house do not. You bring it home to the bedroom and even the bathroom, where medicine and bleach have replaced candle light. Or, as Tony once noted, Your wife becomes your nurse.

Even before serious decline, intimacy changes.

I'm thinking of a recent fundraiser walk for Alzheimer's, Tony's first, with all of us gathering in the hall before the start. It is crowded, and Tony doesn't know where the washroom is. I say I'll show him, and as we step through the doors and into a sea of people, I take his arm. He tells me, Let go! and yanks it away. The message is clear: Don't touch me.

Now I know that if, for instance, you see a sight-impaired person about to cross the street, you ask, first, if they need help rather than grab their arm. But taking Tony's arm is an act of affection. This is my husband, not a stranger. And yet. In this hall full of Alzheimer's supporters and sufferers, where he is confronted by his greatest fear and in turn recoils from everything about it, he is a stranger to all around him, even to me.

This is what Alzheimer's does to a marriage. This is silent grief.

In some ways, Tony has taken the final diagnosis in stride. Cinda agrees with me. He has already acknowledged the presence of Alzheimer's. However, he has still kept his condition secret from many former co-workers and friends. That is its own form of grief, as can be seen in this email he sends me:

> This is the draft of a letter I wrote to a friend I used to see regularly, but hadn't really talked with for about four years. We recently met on the street and promised to get together with some other friends that meet regularly at a nearby pub.
>
> I thought it might provide a glimpse into what my "new life" is about.
>
> Oh, by the way, it was never sent.
>
> Hey:
>
> So nice of you to move so quickly on this, and apologies for the long the delay.
>
> When we bumped into each other a couple of weeks ago and talked about this, I wasn't really thinking well. And now I am hesitant. Here is why:

For one, I don't drink any more, except for a small glass of wine at dinner. I'm still working at this, which means I'm a real downer in a pub.

Also, I rarely read newspapers any more. Yes, I know I worked in them for many years and once was the ultimate newspaper reporter, reveling in the speed of it all, the witnessing of events great and small, the meeting and sometimes befriending interesting, and occasionally life-changing people such as such as Terry Fox, the Queen, world leaders and rebels. But those days are over now, and I don't much like newspapers now. Simply, the life — once so exotic and enlivening, now seems irrelevant and silly.

Because of that, and, probably my age I'm a dud on that score. Instead, I have become one of those people who spends their later years philosophizing, learning, and experiencing the joys of "free thinking" — ie just following your interests and, occasionally, applying them to your own life. It is the longed-dreamed-of life of the amateur scholar.

So I spend most of my time these days philosophizing, or at least reading and studying philosophy, which to most people is the most boring subject on earth. So I am trying hard not to be a philosophy bore who goes around quoting Epictetus as examples of how they should live their life. I try very hard now not to give my opinion on anything and everything and quietly let other, younger people, insist that they know everything there is to know.

Also I have been seriously studying everything I can about things like Buddhism, which I find very peaceful, and other s things (one considered woo-woo) things like meditation, etc. (actually, I have become a meditation freak, which makes me doubly boring.). I even belong to a Buddhist Centre where I am studying the Sangha —(which isn't that hard, since I live across the street from it)

So I am now one of those people we used to laugh at long ago because they went around constantly talking about peace and love (but not dope, even thought it's now legal!)

All of this has made me into something of a pariah among normal people who talk about real stuff. I simply don't know what to say. Most of what people talk about these days (i.e Trump, work, TV ,etc. etc. ) tends to go right over my head. (literally, and many times thankfully).

Next, and more practically, I'm still paying off debts from my disastrous foray into business, life, etc. which doesn't really have anything to do with this, except that I am on a pretty tight (self-imposed) leash when it comes to spending money, especially on something like booze.

Lastly, and most important, I think.....

I should let you know that I have Alzheimer's Disease, which really changes .... well... everything.

It's early but still there, and very slowly advancing i.e. my spelling, and talking, once my specialty, is is getting dreadful. Worse I am constantly forgetting who people I haven't seen or talked with for a while are. Sometimes I can't even remember who they are, although that might be because I met hundreds of people in my life and work, and can't be expected to remember them all.

I console myself on this score by telling myself that most people don't have anything to say anyway or just aren't as important to me as they once were because they aren't in my life now.

I also have to be careful about revealing this, because some people when they hear this go through various versions of recoil involving surprise, fear, and confusion about how to act. Some just talk louder or talk very simply and slowly, like that is going to help. Some just remember they had something pressing to do and just disappear as if it's catching.

So I try to keep it quiet. I don't go around with a big letter A on my chest. I try not to drool and poop my pants when I am with others — the Alzheimer's drugs tend to affect the bowels, so you have to compensate with other drugs or better scheduling. (just another humiliation created by my "friend" Al, (as I now call my doppelganger in order to make him less scary.)

But lately people have been noticing that I'm sometimes kind of weird, i.e. repeating myself, forgetting what they said, etc. I don't really care about it — I have adopted the general attitude that shit happens—the modern version of a central Stoic philosophy (also very Buddhist by the way.)

However, Al, as I call my now doppelganger, does seem to bother or embarrass or anger some others. So I try to remain quiet instead of being my usual talky self — very much still a work in progress, as I am constantly reminded.

Instead I now have a kind of bookish, pleasant but bland, persona, much like when I was very young. . Of course, that might be a complete fantasy on my part but I'm sticking to it.

I may be forgetful and a little weird now, but I'm not stupid.

When I point out to Tony that this book will prove a much larger "coming out" than a letter, he agrees, but says that at least then he won't have to answer any questions from such friends. The book will do that for him.

I have mentioned before the need for repeated email reminders in order to get Tony to respond, and that for the latter part of 2018 Tony stopped emailing me entirely. However, he was still responding just before his birthday in March, when a comment of mine, in continuation of our previous email exchange, inadvertently brought up the subject of death.

March 12, 2018

I am glad of two things. First, that continuing the project on my own, and only if need be, is still okay with you. We simply don't know what the future might bring and if there is one thing you and your family have taught me it is to be practical. The other thing I'm glad of is your continued emphasis on being calm and at peace. You actively seek to enjoy each day and I'm sure some of that has rubbed off on me. I suppose we have to give some credit to approaching spring and longer daylight hours, don't we? There is nothing like sunlight to boost spirits.

March 12, 2018

Again, some interesting starting points here — or maybe I should say some diverging continuing points, or maybe some philosophical points, which is where my real interest lies.

As I look at turning 69 (hell let's just call it 70 since at that age, the difference between the two is so minimal as to be almost non-existent. Seventy is only 12 months away, which is chickenfeed as they used to say down on the farm (somewhere, probably in the backwoods of Cliche' County).

I believe what I said, or thought, anyway, was I had maybe 10 years left, which, from this current viewpoint is quite a while. That's a lot of time in which I might be able to actually accomplish something lasting, leave some kind of legacy — even if it's, "well, he was kind of an interesting guy (the famous Canadian back-in in full form)" — before I turn into dust or vegetable-added sustenance biscuits, or whatever they will be doing with dead bodies in the crowded future (why waste all that valuable protein? Soylent Green is Us!).

As my every-practical mother said (I'm paraphrasing, her's was more colourful, had something to do with the turnip pile), why make a big and expensive to-do about it all. I'll be gone and won't care?

So, as for that, I say, just get rid of me. Throw me in the river. Or if you want spectacle, put me on a pyre, throw on some gasoline, and torch me (Sounds very Viking-ish, or ancient....hmmmm cool!).

As for continuing the project on your own: Of course. It would be only half done if you don't, and a bad half at that. All, you'd have is my meandering, my bad jokes and cracks and the occasional boredom-driven depression. Jeez, who would want to read that? (how to sink a book, 101).

Interesting that you noticed the peace-and-calm approach I am taking. Kind of differentI've been working on that for some time, but never got anywhere, mostly because of my personality (creative, wandering, unruly and gadfly-ish, euphoric or depressed).

You mentioned the things we talked about in the kitchen during one of our heart-to-hearts (which I really enjoy, by the way — ever note that they are almost always in the kitchen? Hmmmm, that says something but I'm not sure what).

I believe I have pretty well done with the first one — coming to terms with ...uh ...fading.

March 19, 2018

Egads, no, I didn't mean when you are "gone" as in end of life. I'm glad we are having these written discussions so we can clarify any misconceptions — this one is my fault, entirely. I should have repeated the initial question because I know that end of life has been on your mind lately. You list some gory "end" options here, including Soylent Green and even your mother's turnip pile! All done with humour, of course, and in fact you've never actually stated your true preference. (For the record, I would like my ashes sprinkled in Stanley Park near one of the beaches, so that part of me would stay on land and the rest be washed out into the Pacific.)

But back to the topic at hand, no I was referring to a future point when you might lose interest in the project. This could come about for many reasons, including being distracted by something else, but mostly I was thinking of the disease itself (Alzheimer's) and the possibility that you might find the editing and restructuring phase overwhelming, as you have in the recent past with some book-length

projects. At any rate, it's good to know you wouldn't be upset if I had to take over the project, especially if it was half
done. Don't think your half would be a bad half, either. Both
of us are scribbling as we go. We don't know where this writing is going to lead us, and that's part of the journey, isn't it?

After this exchange, I let the silence stretch out, not bothering
with the usual reminders. I was occupied with weaving the correspondence, much of it from 2017, into an overall narrative. However,
I showed Tony the resulting draft, and he then became eager to contribute more and began writing again, as upcoming pages will reveal.

We have spent all of Tony's sixth decade searching for answers, and
now the questions and the decade have ended. It's 2019, and he
has reached the age where it isn't all that shocking for a person to
be showing signs of dementia, though I can imagine many seventy-
year-olds objecting to that statement.

At UBC, the neurologist gives him the usual test. His score is
nineteen out of thirty, just one point lower than last time, but a
momentous point. He has hit the teens, and there is no climbing
back up. He is shown the three animals and can't name the third
one, a hippopotamus, calling it a pig with a big, funny nose. He
can count back from one hundred by sevens well enough, until he
forgets how many he is supposed to count back by. He has zero
recall on the string of five words.

He has received his HandyCard, a card that gives him access to
TaxiSavers. With them, he takes the taxi to Paul's Club when I have
to work. This move became necessary during the confusion and
crowding of morning rush hour on transit. One time, a mentally
ill man approached the jammed platform and, of all of us there,
chose Tony to grab by the shoulders and shake to demand a watch.

What had this man seen in Tony? A vulnerability in his expression?

Another time, I stepped off the train at my stop to see that Tony, instead of stepping aside, stood right in the middle of the open doorway. The surge of riders knocked him backwards.

Now, he arrives in style by cab on Tuesdays.

The HandyCard also gives him access to the HandyDART, a mini-bus for those with disabilities. He was not ready to take it that first year, and only recently, approaching his third year, did that change. It came with familiar objections and rants, as each change does. I listened, and Paul's Club listened, and we offered alternatives: he could take the HandyDART back home while I would take him there by train. Then, just as suddenly, the objections stopped and now he willingly climbs aboard.

He also wears a MedicAlert tag around his neck that is engraved with *Tony — Alzheimer's*. At first, he didn't want to wear it, but now he puts it on without being asked. Somewhere along the way, he reached acceptance of the need for it.

We try home support, with the expected first-time bumps. I learn that I should write out instructions, as support workers won't necessarily know ahead of time what Tony's issues are, and that I should add half an hour to the allotted time as they can arrive late.

When I introduce one of the workers to Tony, she turns to me and asks where our father is. It takes me a heartbeat to realize what she means. I point to Tony's retreating back and tell her that he is the person she would be looking after.

He is so young, she says.

Yes.

Tony didn't see the need for a worker, but as with all other stages of his situation, as mentioned, he has come to accept this as well.

On a beautiful spring day, as his sixth decade closes, we celebrate his seventieth birthday, and hear from many that he is in top form and just like the old Tony. His sisters are there, his nephew and son and daughter-in-law and grandchildren and their dad, his friends, his wife.

I suppose it is enough that those in my support group know that for him to get there in that shape I had to ensure he took a nap and then a shower, got dressed in the clothes I laid out, and then got into the cab I booked. All he had to do when he arrived was eat, drink, and be merry. That has always been his forte, and we are fortunate that it is, still.

Cinda notes, however, that within days he is struggling. She has stayed over to give me a much-appreciated break. Without them, I'd collapse. While I'm away, though, she has a medical emergency that requires her son, Stephen, to rush them to Emergency late at night. There, Tony gets away on them, which they only realize when they hear nurses yelling about privacy and confidentiality.

Tony, ever the inquisitive reporter, has forgotten himself and gone behind the counter of the nurses' station. He is looking up at the screens, calling out interesting patient information to his sister and nephew, clearly in violation of the aforementioned privacy and confidentiality regulations. Stephen has to dart over to explain things.

The next day, Stephen drives his mom to an early-morning specialist's appointment, and from there takes Tony to Paul's Club. The following morning Cinda has surgery for a detached retina, and Tony spends an extra day at Paul's Club, which I arrange, long-distance. Again, Nita and Michael Levy come to our rescue.

I arrive home to find Garth and Stephen overseeing things while Cinda and Tony are just waking from a long sleep, weary from their own private ordeals.

Later, Cinda tells me that, unlike in past visits, Tony repeatedly asked her the same questions, was difficult to get moving in the early morning, forgot that he must get moving because she had important medical appointments, and showed general confusion. She had reached the same point the gerontologist had, finally seeing him as I have been seeing him at home, and for some time.

I am away for only four nights. On Cinda's previous visits, he didn't have to do anything other than get in the car she was driving and go to a movie or a restaurant. This time, there was an emergency, and he had to do something, including stay up late at night, get up early, follow new directions, and act quickly.

Cinda agrees that the disruptions caused Tony a lot of problems, adding that several times he told her that his routine was off. She apologized to him for having to change things. A routine would have caged the wandering spirit of the old Tony. Now, he needs it. Sudden change threatens his ability to cope.

At the end of this long decade, Tony is all too aware of the many shifts and sudden turns in his life. Sometimes he is angry and sometimes he is bewildered, as though he can't quite believe it's happening to him. At other times, as in the following, he traces back the changes, looking for those first signs, the proof that, yes, it is indeed happening and, most important, it likely was happening for many years previously. The words spring from the conversation he and I had earlier about the purpose of this project, and the email from me in which I had quoted him saying that no one thinks they might have Alzheimer's. I sent him a note later, letting him know where I was in the manuscript, suggesting: Why not put that line here and expand upon it? Three paragraphs, perhaps. More, if you feel like it. It's a line that reverberates, has resonance.

So that's exactly what he did.

I can tell you right now it never occurs to anyone that they might have Alheimer's disease.

They're tired; they drink too much; life is too fast; there is too much to do; it's the weather, just a brain cramp, and probably a dozen or more other explanations for the increasing incidence of memory gaps , behavior foibles, and short zone-outs that they are experiencing with some regularity.

Yes, perhaps, if they are older, they might have vaguely considered it, largely because they hear about it everywhere — in the news, on television, from conversations at get-togethers, during conversations where people joke about "senior's moments." But that's all out there somewhere, not on their radar.

I know because I used them all, and a few other creative descriptions to explain the strange memory blips that were happening to me too often to ignore or explain away. It couldn't be the Alzheimer's, the dreaded black cloud they said might be lurking in the future for all of us who were now being called "early seniors", meaning we weren't young, but we weren't old either. We were "mature" (yeah, that's it, mature!)

And certainly, it couldn't be me, — the guy with the flypaper brain, the one everybody else in the newsroom turned to for information or spelling, or plain old random knowledge. I was the human notebook, for god's sake. Heck, I even remembered birthdays — most of the time.

But there came a point where all my explanations didn't work. I was forgetting things regularly, little things like someone's name whom I hadn't seen for a while but should have known, or a directions that I had followed some time ago but now were a bit foggy. Increasingly, I had to search for words or names or other information that should have been retrievable after a little thought. It was clear my memory was failing, and I didn't know why.

Was it all the sports and other injuries I suffered as a teen and a young man? My wild and crazy period when I roamed around North America and Europe, "learning" about life by leaping into it, often, I admit, with the help of a few banned substances? Maybe it was a result of some of the brawling I did in my young manhood, not out of desire, but more because circumstances I had found myself in required it.

Then there were the years of struggle and constant depression that seemed to paper my early path into the straight life.

Could it have been the journalist's disease — delving into human tragedy and pain constantly, and then drinking to "shake it off." It was that kind of life, but I I believed I learned to cope, and that all the mental and physical injuries healed quickly (I thought). I never believed I had a drinking problem, but it was pretty steady.

Maybe it was continual bumping up against tragedy that had been my specialty. I was the ultimate viewer of the downside of the human condition, the "hack" they sent out to talk to the family when someone died, whether naturally or, most often, unnaturally; the author or famous person who had a tragic or uplifting story to tell; the great empath who could instantly take on someone else's worst troubles and sooth them somewhat. Sometimes they would even ask me to help them with arrangements and I almost did it .... until I remembered the journalist's code to see and tell the story .... not be part of it.

And now I was living the ultimate irony ..... I was the story.

# ALZHEIMER'S BY THE NUMBERS

There is an expression in the news business: Does this story have legs? In other words, does it have staying power, will it make it to the end?

I picture that etched glass, with patterns of brain cells stretching out across the expanse of windows. Legs? This story has tentacles, and they reach well beyond the life of its main character.

Tony's nephews and niece, and their children and their children's children, as well as his stepson, whose grandmother was similarly afflicted, are all wrapped up in the outcome. So are my sister's children. Perhaps members of your family are, too.

Each of them, ready for the longshot that is life, must observe us and wonder: Will it be me, next? Will I be the one in our family to succumb? Or will our generation be the one to defeat this disease? Will we be the ones to step into the future without fear of that future, to know that whatever calamity greets us, we can at least be assured that our minds will be intact, our futures solid, and that our pasts, those precious memories that form who we are, will remain until the end?

I certainly hope so.

Alzheimer's at any age is life-changing, but the younger the person, the more life that is irreparably changed. An online article from the Mayo Clinic begins with the headline: "Young-Onset Alzheimer's: When Symptoms Begin Before Age 65." Note that the focus of the article is on when symptoms begin, not when a diagnosis is given. It is an important distinction, as it can take years to get a diagnosis. "When Alzheimer's begins in middle age," the article continues, "misdiagnosis may be more likely."

The terms *young-* and *early-onset* are often used interchangeably. I prefer to use young-onset, as early-onset is easily confused for the early stages of Alzheimer's. Also, young-onset emphasizes an important point that I will expand upon shortly, which is how many years back changes to the brain can occur.

Most people with young-onset Alzheimer's develop symptoms of the disease in their forties and fifties. While Tony was dubbed the absent-minded professor in his forties, it was in his fifties that he began to show clear indicators: loss of interest in his job, loss of interest in the garden, increased forgetfulness, temper flare-ups, depression. There were the beginnings of stove and other mishaps during those years, and then, in early 2011, when he was sixty-one, a fall that marked the point of no return to normal cognitive function.

Tony is taking part in a couple of research studies at UBC's Alzheimer's clinic, one that looks at changes over a five-year period, and the other a shorter one that observes visual connections. One day, I asked a researcher in the five-year study where he would place Tony: under young- or late-onset. He asked me to review the events that I have just written about, and then remarked that the prescription of Aricept for Tony in 2015 marked the time of his diagnosis. In 2015 Tony was sixty-six. I nodded, and said, But what of the symptoms, as I have just outlined them, that go back for many more years?

Now he nodded. He is on the borderline, he said.

In other words, Tony will not be included in any research numbers that any of us might read in future reports on young-onset Alzheimer's disease. By this reckoning, which creates a cut-off at the taking of a pill rather than the setting of kitchen fires, he does not exist in those statistics.

I asked the same question of the neurologist, who also placed Tony on the borderline, noting the fall in early 2011, when he was sixty-one, and adding that while the cut-off is often set at age sixty-five, he considered the younger group of young-onset to be age sixty and under.

We have friends and acquaintants who have been struck with this disease at a younger age. Elise's husband, Steve, was fifty-three. John Mann was slightly younger and would die in November 2019, at age fifty-seven.

Tony was simply younger than is the case in the more typical late-onset Alzheimer's. As I noted above, in his fifties Tony was showing signs of cognitive trouble. Along with memory issues, he began showing visuospatial problems. Research published in the *Journal of Alzheimer's Disease* in 2010 under the title, "Early- Versus Late-Onset Alzheimer's Disease: More Than Age Alone," found that while memory loss is typical of Alzheimer's disease, non-memory presentations especially occur in patients with early-onset AD.

In particular, visuospatial dysfunction appeared in one third of the test subjects who had young-onset, but in only 6 percent of the late-onset.

Tony worked hard at fighting all the symptoms once they arrived in full force at age sixty-one. His very determination to fight could be the reason the disease's progress has been slow. Or it could be just luck.

While there has been considerable research on all forms of dementia, more is needed, and especially in the area of young-onset Alzheimer's disease. I have heard several doctors and professionals say they are observing an increased incidence of young-onset, and whether this will be supported by research remains to be seen.

It could be that in the past, the diagnosis for patients was delayed, as it was in Tony's case, and that the symptoms had appeared at a much younger age than the one formally documented. Now that medical professionals and family members are becoming more aware, they are recognizing the symptoms sooner. Hence the increase.

In Australia and the United States, records show that 5 percent of those diagnosed with Alzheimer's have young-onset. In Canada, according to the Canadian Institute for Health Information, it's 3 percent. Are we doing something wonderful here, or is it a matter of how the numbers are interpreted? *The Provincial Guide to Dementia Care in British Columbia* cites 8 percent, while the Alzheimer Society of Canada puts the number between 2 to 8 percent. In all likelihood, these numbers will change. In the minister's message in the recent document "A Dementia Strategy for Canada: Together We Aspire," the Honourable Ginette Petitpas Taylor acknowledged, "We know that there are more than 419,000 Canadians aged 65 and older diagnosed with dementia, but this is only part of the story. This number does not capture those under the age of 65 with a diagnosis of dementia and those who, possibly due to stigma or other barriers, remain undiagnosed."

In the above articles, some of the statistics refer to young- and late-onset dementia as opposed to Alzheimer's disease; however, Alzheimer's is the most common of the dementias. Of note as well is frontotemporal dementia, which can be misdiagnosed as young-onset Alzheimer's. It tends to strike at younger ages, forty-five being typical, but behavioural changes, more than memory issues, are some of the early indicators.

The patient with the unlucky distinction of being the first one diagnosed with what would be called Alzheimer's disease would also, by today's medical standards, be considered to fall under young-onset.

Auguste Deter was only fifty-one years of age when she was seen by Dr. Alois Alzheimer in 1901. When she died just shy of her fifty-sixth birthday, her brain was found to have the plaques and tangles that are considered to be typical of the disease. Mario Mendez, the director of the Neurobehavior Clinic at the David Geffen School of Medicine at UCLA, noted that with the observation of similar cognitive decline in all age groups, "investigators subsequently broadened the diagnosis of AD to include the much more common late-onset AD (LOAD)." In recent years, the main focus of interest and research has been on LOAD; however, like Auguste Deter, patients with EOAD remain an important and impactful subgroup of patients with this disorder.

In other words, there are so many more in that late-onset category that Alzheimer's disease came to be associated with the senior age group, but the discovery of it began with young-onset.

Tony's choice of *Four Umbrellas* as the title of this book is more accurate than he might have imagined, since the idea of the umbrella is useful for defining the disease itself. *Dementia* is an umbrella term that includes Alzheimer's disease; and *Alzheimer's* itself is an umbrella term for at least four forms of the disease: the familial form of young-onset, which I will describe in more detail, and which strikes the very young; the under-sixty-five form of young-onset, which our neurologist said should really be used for those under sixty; the over sixty-five, called late- or older-onset, which comprises the largest numbers; and then the borderline group to which Tony belongs.

But then, I'm no scientist, just an observer. There are likely more or different categories that medical teams have noted.

Family physicians and ER doctors are on the front lines — they are the first experts we see. It is essential that they familiarize themselves with the signs of dementia, regardless of the age of the patient. Amazing, isn't it, that I have to write that and that governments such as Canada's have to draw up strategies calling for greater confidence among primary care practitioners in diagnosing dementia early, when Auguste Deter and her doctor, Alois Alzheimer, paved the way for early recognition over one hundred years ago.

Doctors, in general, need to pay more attention to the family members who step forward with concerns. If these concerns are repeated and extended over time, and if they worsen, for heaven's sake, stop hesitating and order up the tests immediately, not just the MoCA but an MRI and the intensive, day-long memory tests.

Had Tony been given the MRI after his trip to Emergency in early 2011, when he was sixty-one, where would he be placed on the Alzheimer's scale? And does it matter?

Yes.

Getting a diagnosis sooner is important to the family that must make financial and other arrangements, as well as to the person whose brain is suddenly and inexplicably not functioning as it once was. Jobs are lost when this happens, friends and family are offended, and isolation deepens. I keep hearing how expensive an MRI is, but what is the cost to society as a whole when an illness goes untreated? When unexplained changes in behaviour lead to marital breakdown, and families and friendships fall apart because neither party understands the reason for the changes? Or when a portion of the population must give up work to provide unpaid hours of caregiving? What happens to those caregivers' career aspirations, to their potential contributions to commerce, education, the arts? Their absence is society's loss.

Getting a diagnosis sooner is important to science. The numbers need to be adjusted to reflect just how many people under the age of sixty-five are struggling with the disease. To get an accurate picture of things, it's important that special efforts be made to include information on marginalized populations, since such things as impoverishment and poor education are likely barriers to obtaining a timely diagnosis. As well, there are structural barriers to obtaining an early diagnosis. The separation by age of the population suffering from Alzheimer's, for example. Why the arbitrary boundary of age sixty-five? Is it because that's retirement age, when pensions and escalating medical costs begin? Or because that's where government funding for research kicks in? Consider the person diagnosed at the age of seventy, who has likely been showing signs for many years before, with brain changes as far back as twenty years, to age fifty, when he or she was holding down a job and paying off a mortgage and raising a family. My mother, for instance.

This is not an old person's disease. The same can be said of cancer and many other diseases, but bears repeating with this disease in particular.

Any time you hear of someone being diagnosed with Alzheimer's, ask the age, then subtract twenty years, and if you get a number that shocks you, repeat after me: This is not an old person's disease.

Am I wrong to focus on the number twenty? It occurs to me. After all, the study I have in mind states changes to the brain had been found to take place *up to* twenty years previously. Perhaps I was guilty of, if not exaggerating then emphasizing the larger number.

I hit the computer to look up the numbers again. The research, published in *Lancet Neurology* in December 2012, looked at an extended family in Colombia that carried a gene for the young-onset form of Alzheimer's. They were ideal study candidates because of the familial connection and therefore high likelihood of the disease showing up in the subjects — 50 percent of the offspring go on to develop the disease, called familial Alzheimer's disease (FAD). Members with the gene, the study said, tend to show memory problems in their mid-forties and full-blown Alzheimer's in their fifties. The scientists discovered that many young people, some as young as eighteen, had changes in their brain, blood, and nervous systems that presaged the onset of Alzheimer's decades later.

As I was scanning down the screen, I found many more articles citing detection twenty years earlier — so many articles, in fact, that it was overwhelming. There's even a term for those early signs before diagnosis: *preclinical Alzheimer's disease.* I then caught sight of a headline that had me scrolling back and reading: it was a reference to a study out of Johns Hopkins University that allowed scientists to look at people over a period of twenty and thirty years before they presented clinical symptoms. These study subjects were forty years of age and older, and had a family history of the disease. The article doesn't state if this means they carried the gene for FAD. I gather they didn't, because of the 290 subjects, only eighty-one would go on to develop MCI or dementia, and that is notably less than 50 percent. What was remarkable, however, was that when researchers looked at spinal fluid levels for a type of molecule linked to Alzheimer's, called tau proteins, they found that there was a significant increase in the levels of these proteins over time, and that this buildup started almost thirty-five years before symptoms developed in those eighty-one subjects.

Back in Colombia, the scientists studying the extended family are looking at other family members ages seven to seventeen to see whether brain changes occur at an even younger age.

Seven years old. I don't even need to say it, do I?

The second study Tony is taking part in looks at visual and verbal responses. There has been a documented connection between Alzheimer's and a part of the brain where ocular function is centred, and these tests hope to show that Alzheimer's can be seen in a simple eye exam, which would make early detection that much more feasible.

When one member of the research team heard about our book, she asked if I knew about the study on writers and Alzheimer's, and mentioned the novelist Iris Murdoch. We were on the phone, and I'm sure I gasped. I had enjoyed John Bayley's memoir *Elegy for Iris*. It was published the same year as "Not Me," and I must have read it before the final edit because I mention her in the story. Earlier, I wrote that I can't say for sure this book wasn't my idea. This is because, in describing the project to others, publishers included, I have said that I have always wondered about Murdoch's thoughts as her dementia progressed and how she might have written about the experience in *Elegy*, had she had the opportunity. *Four Umbrellas* would give Tony that chance. So perhaps it was my idea, with Tony quickly jumping on board. At any rate, I told the researcher I would like to see the paper, and the next day my inbox contained a copy of the 2011 study out of the University of Toronto.

The authors of "Longitudinal Detection of Dementia Through Lexical and Syntactic Changes in Writing: A Case Study of Three British Novelists" found that it is probable that Agatha Christie suffered from the onset of undiagnosed Alzheimer's while writing her last novels, but that Iris Murdoch showed symptoms much earlier in her career. The findings indicate she "exhibited a 'trough' of relatively impoverished vocabulary and syntax in her writing in her late 40s and 50s that presaged her later dementia." Murdoch was diagnosed with Alzheimer's at around age seventy-five, which means her brain was showing changes over twenty-five years earlier. (The third novelist, P.D. James, aged "healthily.")

The project hasn't stopped there, and will be expanded in the future to include more subjects and broaden its scope, not just in literary text but in ordinary functional daily writing. It concludes with a note that is both tantalizing and intimidating. "For future generations, who are already building a lifetime archive of electronic communications, the availability of past text for eventual diagnosis will not be a problem." Indeed. Think of our hastily hammered out emails, texts, and tweets, with all of their typos and missing words, prime pickings for scientific scrutiny.

Well. Studies take time, and Tony's ocular one has just begun. The findings might not be available for years, and whatever they find, it will be too late for us. The results of the five-year study will be further along, yet. Tony is taking part for the sake of those future generations.


Until there is better news, I have one message for spouses and children: Speak up during medical appointments. Don't be shy. Document the changes you are noticing, those early warning signs, then write them up and bring them to the next appointment. Email them to the doctor ahead of time if you want the concerns to arise naturally in that session. Ask for copies of doctors' notes from each appointment.

Seek a second opinion if you feel your concerns are being dismissed.

Push hard for an MRI.

Then go to your own doctor and cry all over the floor if you have to. You need help, too, because it's a very long road ahead of you. Join support groups and share your knowledge. Keep in mind, and remind all those around you, that whether it's a parent or partner you're caring for, that caring stops if you aren't being looked after, too.

Tony and I wrote *Four Umbrellas* not only to understand what has happened to us, but also to offer insight to anyone facing a similar journey. We have shared our experiences to the best of our ability so that others can not only trace the trajectory and compare, but also consider those early warning signs that are vital to an early diagnosis, and yet so often go unnoticed or are misinterpreted.

This book is our way of saying to all: Pay attention.


Tony has always described Alzheimer's as a fogginess. Recently, however, he has begun describing something different, a custard that coats the brain, he says.

I hustle him into his office to write it down.

What follows is a description that only someone like Tony could write. He made his living with words. And yes, there is that other thing. We can put statistics aside for the moment and take in the words of someone who is an expert in this particular area. This is what it feels like to have Alzheimer's disease:

> Four Umbrellas brain blob, An Alzheimers horror vision.
>
> Some times I can feel themt, almost. The dying brain cells
>
> I'll wake up and think, something happened over night ... like, inside my head, a big crust of gooey meringue is creeping along from the sides of my forehead along both temples.
>
> That's probably because I've seen images of a brain with alzheimers ... that's what I'm picturing.
>
> What's bothering me about it though, is that as it moves, crushing everything everything it touches, there's this wasteland left behind.
>
> A nuclear blast zone, where everything that was once there is now dead.

I know the picture comes from my mind — and likely from some images that I have seen — but it is positively frightening.

This is real; that death creep is going on in my own head.

I am watching my own slow death. And there is nothing I can do to stop it.

In fact, it is almost worse, because I will not be dead.

I will just be shell, a body without a purpose except to stay ahem-alive-ahem.

This is a glimpse into my future: a mass of dead or dying flesh that was once a human being. No joy, no sorrow, no laughter, no past, no future.

Nothing that makes us human.

# ONE HUNDRED DAYS AND COUNTING

We begin 2020 full of marvel at the bigness of the number, the passage of time, the prospect of this book reaching the public in the fall. Within a few short weeks, everything changes.

A former student of mine dies, and between his funeral and the wake, my brother dies. These two deaths strike me as no others before, coming close together as they have, but also because I had known these men as boys, and it is the boys I mourn, the lives that could have been. In both cases, and for different reasons, their hearts have given out, and is there anything more symbolically charged than that?

Tony and I had been to visit my brother just three weeks before, bringing him food and money, as Tom was feeling ill but refused to go to a hospital. We have to return, now, to clear things from his apartment, and Mary Beth helps me that first night. We worry about what we might uncover in there, but I'm unable to find masks in any stores, only medical gloves, and we put those on right away. Tom lived a reclusive life in a single room, and the bed where he died looms in that cramped space as we bag and bundle for several hours. Garth stays at home with Tony that first night, and then the three of us spend the rest of the weekend at Tom's — more bagging and stacking. Garth and I are kept on our toes, as Tony sets things on that bed, or sits himself on that bed, or touches items best left untouched. Garbage. Soiled clothing. Cigarette butts. The bathroom. I tell our neighbour Mike about the stack of record albums, as he has a vinyl collection. A friend was supposed to pick them up but didn't show. I warn Mike about the state of the place, but he drops by anyway, and we are relieved to have one more task completed.

Back home, flowers and cards begin to arrive, the phone rings repeatedly. Each time, Tony asks me, Did someone die?

More than once I shut the bathroom door to have a cry.

The business of death takes time, so it's a couple of weeks before arrangements can be made. Pam flies down and we scatter our brother's ashes. We go for dinner one night and are surprised at how empty the restaurant is. In the parking lot, we run into some neighbours. There is handshaking — still — and condolences.

The next day, Prime Minister Trudeau urges all Canadians abroad to come home and those who are here to stay home. The national shutdown of all but essential businesses begins. I am only partially aware of the impending pandemic, being absorbed in what has been going on in my personal life.

That same day, I get an email from Paul's Club saying that it has closed temporarily. I also learn that I have been laid off at the treatment centre, which has suspended its arts program workshops due to COVID-19. Oddly, this doesn't send me into an emotional tailspin, even though this job had brought a sense of balance to my life. Everyone I know has lost something in the pandemic, and that in itself levels the loss.

It's only then, thanks to the advice of Garth and Stephen, that I race out to stock up on non-perishable items, as apparently many people had been doing for some time. I want to order groceries online but each time I try there are no open spaces. Garth, however, helps me set up an Amazon account, and so I'm able to order such things as giant sacks of cat litter and packages of printing paper.

After Garth's visit, we communicate with him by phone or video. We meet our nephew once for a Sunday walk, but the crowds are so thick we vow not to try that again. Friends stay at home, too, of course, so it's just Tony and me. However, a simple wave or shouted greeting from neighbours in and about our small building is comforting and creates a sense of community.

I take Tony shopping with me once for last-minute items I have forgotten. We still have no masks so use scarves instead. The shelves are empty and the line-ups long. Repeatedly, anxious to move ahead, Tony pushes the cart forward, hitting my leg. Each time, I ask him to stop pushing, and finally I suggest he wait at the other end of the line until I bring the cart through. I think I'm saying it nicely, but I look up to see a man behind us glaring at me.

There is no longer home support, except for emergencies. So, yes, I am probably cranky. But do I even want someone in our home who has been tending to ill people in several other homes that day? I try for more patience.

Until online shopping spots open up, Tony and I learn to be content on a diet of spaghetti and chili and more spaghetti. Neighbours are kind and offer to pick up items if we run out. Our dear niece Uche calls to say she and her beau will reschedule their Toronto wedding; the publisher emails to advise us this book's release will be postponed. Our lives grow quiet.

I am busy, though. Each day begins with emails and chores. Tony and I go for a walk to give both of us a break from being cooped up in an apartment. The fresh air and exercise help to calm Tony, and he then sleeps for two hours after lunch while I hammer away on the keyboard, finishing up the last of the revisions. Or I read a book.

For the first month or so, it's an adventure. As most of us do, we take in more virtual events. An art gallery lecture. Poetry readings. A couple of friends have work in anthologies that launch virtually. I belong to a novelists' salon group, and its next session is virtual as is my mindfulness care group. Our strata meetings, too, have moved to video format.

Closer to May, Tony and I begin to putter in the garden on the rooftop patio. Leighton next door works as a gardener and is a great source of over-the-fence advice and information. In the evenings, Tony and I watch movies or a couple of episodes of a series. Eventually, we get an online shopping order in. We discover the extended winter farmers' market, too, with well-marked spots for physical distancing, another chance to get out and breathe fresh air.

It's reassuring that everyone else is going through a similar situation, but living through a pandemic while simultaneously living with dementia is a different kind of nightmare. There is no relief from the repetition, the missing items, especially the masks we eventually find and buy, the reminders to wash those hands, the arguments when Tony feels he doesn't need to.

I'm seeing those snakes under the bed again. I also see that "Not Me" was my own early version of those snakes. I predicted our future twenty years ago, and that future is now, with the added impact of the pandemic.

As I write this, it's been over one hundred days since the first case of COVID-19 was diagnosed on the West Coast. There has been a great deal of suffering everywhere, and death. However, the curve — as the experts call it — seems to be flattening here, and there are plans for a gradual easing of restrictions, here and elsewhere. Our book is back on for a fall publication. Things are looking up.

It's good the suspensions of my job and Paul's Club coincided, as I could not have gone to work and left Tony alone. I just hope the two resume at the same time.

Programs at the neighbourhood house also stopped, Tony's column included. He says he has enjoyed staying home. In some ways, he can function within the familiar far better than he can out there in an ever-changing world. The simple routine brings that sense of peace I referred to earlier in this narrative. But in other ways, he is struggling more than ever.

I am brain-weary myself today, awakened at 4 a.m. by the sound of Tony getting up to use the washroom. I watch as he faces into the corner of the bedroom, somehow seeing a toilet where the wicker laundry hamper stands. I am out of bed in a flash and steering him across the hall to the bathroom.

This is a first. I cannot fall back to sleep. I keep wondering: What next?

After breakfast, Tony and I discuss how his mind is missing the face-to-face stimulation of Paul's Club, despite the online sessions it has begun holding. This is an unexpected consequence of the COVID-19 lockdown: His dementia has worsened because of isolation, and he is socially distant now, in ways we had not imagined.

Minutes later, I am cleaning up the kitchen when Tony returns to say he is having trouble with a password and asks me, What's my mother's maiden name?

I am thrown by his question. This is long-term knowledge. And it's about his mother. But I try to look unperturbed, wiping the counter and unplugging the kettle as I answer him. He hesitates, and then he asks me, What's her first name?

All this happens in just a four-hour period. On this day that is also, as it turns out, Mother's Day, I am witnessing, in swift succession, a clear progression downward. There is no need for more tests, or more scores, or even more wondering. I have been here before. I know what happens next.

It's Tony's turn to add to this epilogue. He is having trouble writing on his computer, and I suggest, as we have done many times in the past for his neighbourhood house column, that he write his part into the body of an email and send it to me. But that has also become too much for him. Instead, I have him scribble out his thoughts on paper so that I can type them into the manuscript. His handwriting has deteriorated, and we squint over the copy several times to figure out a word or a letter, leaving in any errors we feel are the result not of rushing, but of the disease. Still, when he reads it over, he exclaims at the number of them. Again, I know that such details make this story an important one to tell. But once again, I wish it wasn't ours.

Since June and I initially wrote Four Umbrellas our situation has changeg ... and not always for the better.

My memory has become worse to the point wher conversation, unless they are very important, are forgotten within minutes. Similarly reading & observing and analyzing, which were once my strong points have now all but disappeared.

What is worse is that the relationship June & I had have had for years has changed. What was once a strong partnership has now turned into a form of nursing, which I know is needed, but adimittally annoys me. I miss our old life very, very much.

Further, my writing which I believe was once my strong point is disintegrating. I find it difficult to write anything that is more than a short note. It seems to be an inability to fiocus. This is common when one ages, but I am very aware there I believe that I seem to be ahead of most people when it comes to this disintegration.

Another shok came when a friend of mine who also has Alzheimers was recently put into a facility because his condition worsened. As a result he is constantly trying to "go home" or sits mindlessly for long periods. Of course it is very difficult for me to understand without worrying that this will likely be my future as well.

But enough of this story of woes. There have been some good results. For the most part (I think) I am generally commer now, more willing to accept things, and in a sense am more spiritual. I spend much time now reading about Bhuddism, trying to inculcate some of it's beliefs into my thinking. It's a big change from my formal life but I find it more thoughtful and interesting. I gather that this is not unusual when one has a disease that is forcing one to live in a different world.

# APPENDIX

## Not Me
*by June Hutton*

Originally published in *Other Voices*, Summer 1999

We could be lovers, he with his head caressing blue tiles, me with hands cupped, the shampoo dribbling to my elbows as I reach for those dark curls. Just a strand or two of grey, his skin still tight. But the eyes, the eyes they come unhinged and wander like lost children.

This is what my life has become.

I should be grateful for the moments of clarity when he returns, though he says they are like diving down into the throat of your own reflection. But I am whole, still, reluctant receiver of my mother's benediction.

"You," she told me as I helped with the tulip bulbs, "are resilient." She held the basket and I scooped the papery buds into my hands and scattered them in drifts. "That's why we never worry about you."

Her words meant little then because so soon after she plunged into the sepia glow of the past, calling out names of people I never knew, letting my sister and me slip in and out of her life until we disappeared altogether.

"Who's Jane?" she asked my father after one of her bad spells. I had just arrived clutching half a dozen of the blue-black tulips, and I thought I must be hearing wrong.

"Who's that one?" she later asked a nurse, pointing at my sister who had brought chocolates in the hopes of triggering recognition.

And there it grew, right there, slumped in the bedsheets beside our wild-haired mother: our mutual horror. Which one of us would end up like her? Eating from the cat's dish and crawling out the window in her nightie? Like her mother, and her mother before her?

We never thought how our father must have felt, seeing his bride crumble in his hands like the skins on those tulip bulbs, never considered the agony of bearing witness. We had our own futures to absorb us.

To dodge fate, I found a man who could give me children: to prove I was alive, you see, a sexual creature, capable of giving life. The fact that my mother had had four children with no positive effect whatsoever on her state of mind somehow escaped me. But I had married a husband with foreign roots, a little older, way smarter. Surely that proved a sense of adventure, of broad-mindedness, of resistance, therefore, to dim-wittedness?

My sister went for her B.A., then her M.A., then her Ph.D., to fortify her mind, she said, to keep it sharp and safe from early rot — though she was forced to see her folly when she read about Iris Murdoch who forgot she'd ever written twenty-six novels and who spent her days collecting street garbage that she scattered over the carpet.

My husband laughed at us both. Did we really think birthing and studying would somehow protect us? No one is immune,

Josefus countered. "And where is it stated," he asked, pointing to his temple, "that no men went goofy?"

If only I could take that away, that pointing finger. Our kids would say he'd jinxed himself. But at the time, his words silenced us: Carol with her cup mid-way to her lips; me not even able to pick mine up. Uncle George, we thought at once. Crazy old Uncle George, who slapped the neighbour then ran down the street with his dick dangling out the slit in his pyjamas. He exposed himself for two whole blocks until we caught him.

"Where am I?" he asked my father, as though the strangeness of his deportment was nothing next to the strangeness of the neighbourhood.

And so we began to worry about our brothers and my son. Males from our bloodline. But, really, never with the intensity we worried about ourselves, my daughter, too, because we knew the risk was far greater in women. All the studies said so.

"Jane," my sister scolded one year, grinning, "you sent me two Christmas cards!"

"Oh!" I gushed. "Oh, that. I have two mailing lists. One from the office, one from home. That's how that happened."

But then one Saturday morning a few months later when I'd popped by for coffee, I caught her putting the kettle in the fridge.

"Carol!" I'd cried out.

"Oh, for heaven's sake," she'd laughed. "I was miles away, my Ph.D. defence."

And the sun through the window buttered our skins as though it were any golden day in spring, but we were shaken to see such blunders so early in our lives. How much time did we have? Till forty? Fifty? And who would it strike? Her, or me?

"Why not both of you?" Josefus teased, black eyes sparkling, delighting in mockery, in the irony he saw everywhere.

Oh, the irony. I could eat it up now and spit nails at the mirror. But back then I smiled indulgently at his wit and looked sadly at Carol, who had no husband to teach her such tricks. Maybe solitude would strike her in the back of the head as she bent over her Ph.D. defence. This bantering of wits would prove my salvation.

Carol often said I should stop this sarcasm, this poking fun at what could be our futures.

"You won't think it's so funny, then."

"No," I countered, "because I'll be out of my mind. I won't be thinking anything!"

And I'd laugh because I thought that was what made me resilient.

Unlike her, I didn't finish my English degree. I switched to fine arts before quitting altogether.

It had seemed a wise choice at the time: Travel as the means of education. I had only just met Josefus but he was easily convinced, Europe being his old stomping grounds. We settled on Amsterdam, his favorite city. Drank red wine in the brown cafés and flirted with the notion of living on a canal boat and learning to play guitar. We stayed in a tiny room five floors above Rembrandtsplein with a sliver of a view of dark canal water.

Neither of us got around to playing guitar but we drank coffee while street musicians twanged and sang; we strolled along the paths and bridges. My sister might have been breathing in the dust of books but I was saturated by life: the lilt of different tongues, the tang of raw herring with onion, the musky whiff of his skin.

I could stare at the male shape forever, in the glossy pages of art books, or in the flesh, their arms, their legs, the weight of their sex like plums bending the branches of trees. They fired my imagination the way music or poetry fuelled others. I delighted in their sandpaper chins, large hands and heavy wrists; revelled in the magic of their satiny skins hardening in my hands.

The search stopped at Josefus. Dark-skinned, thickly moustached, he was, I told myself, the perfect means of achieving fruitfulness, of fighting decrepitude. So one night in bed when the stars froze brilliant under the blackest of Amsterdam skies, and he said we'd found our own Starry Night, I looked straight into those dark eyes and said, "Let's get married."

We returned home and had our children quickly. Alexa, then Stephanos, Stevie for short. We bought a house, took the kids camping, got a dog. Life was good, I told myself.

Then I put the kettle in the fridge.

I tried to convince myself I hadn't done it, since I really couldn't remember doing it, but memory is the first thing to go. And I am my sister's sister. She made the same mistake. Maybe Josefus was right: We were both doomed.

Realization dawned slowly. I arrived home one day to find the front door wide open. My face flushed, scalp prickled, heart pounded. I was sure I'd closed it, locked it, but there it was, ajar and offering our belongings to the first thief who passed by. I raced inside to see what had been stolen. To my amazement, nothing. And yet it had sat open for hours, inferring the presence of a careful occupant: Washing the windows, dusting the book shelves, airing the house. Not a mad woman who'd left the door gaping like an astonished mouth behind her. Not me.

So I kept this discovery to myself. Kept my family safe from the terrible knowledge that my mind was slipping. And my humour became a desperate thing, anything, to keep them from suspecting.

One morning at the breakfast table I looked up to see Josefus all ready for work in suit and tie with his fly undone. Here was an opportunity.

"Flying at half-mast?" I cried out, flushing from ears to neck as I scrambled for my next comeback. I reach forward to zip him, laughing. "Don't want the girls at the office —"

"Back off," he shouted, cutting off my quip and twisting to the side.

I stepped forward, uncertain, and he raised his hand as if to hit me.

In her dwindling years my mother had become an escape artist. Unless heavily drugged she broke loose and ran down the halls of the old folks' home, the intravenous tubes and needles, the bandages, flapping from her sides like broken wings, while behind her raced a team of nurses, faces like beets, mouths stretched red with the effort of calling out her name: Ja-a-a-ne!

Just like mine.

Our mother lived until 82. Outlived our bright-minded father by a dozen years. And in her last days, each time the young doctor came by she lifted her nightie over her head and showed him her vagina. Between hysterics Carol and I told each other, "If I ever get like that, take me out in the backyard and shoot me!" Poor Dad, we agreed. Poor old Dad, thank God he never had to see her like that.

Carol was the one person I could have confided in, but something stopped me. The thought that this was just stress? Plain old job pressure? Yes, even in that thought lurked a seed of doubt, waiting to swell and split open, to grow into a monstrous truth that would be far, far worse than my own demise. So I denied it germination, pushed it away, willingly planted the idea that it was me. That way I could still slap it down with laughter, ridicule it into submission. And yet the sight of Josefus fumbling with his fly set my skin creeping along my bones.

Later on the phone Carol would ask who hasn't left their zipper undone, but it was also that look of confusion on his face, so much like our mother's, his raised hand and my now remarkably clear memory of the kettle incident, the open door. The seed had burst open and rolled out into the light, the rank-smelling truth of his decay spilling out. There was no denying it, now. And the humour that had consoled me all these years died swiftly.

The only sounds that day were the ticking of the clock, the clicking of the stove elements as they cooled. He turned on his heel and slammed the door. He knew. How could he not? For years my sister and I had talked of nothing but the telltale signs.

I finished my usual rounds, checked the light switches and TV, the lock on the back door, the windows. But the panic was gone. I moved slowly, ashamed at the relief flooding through me. I remember thinking: It's not me. As though that were somehow better.

Sitting alone at my desk, now, the house finally quiet, I look out the window at the pink light streaking the sky, watch until it turns the lavender of bruises. Last week the trees mocked me with their heavy fruit, fruit that swelled and dripped over thickened trunks. But I couldn't bear to go out there and breathe in the perfume, didn't have the energy to prop up their branches with rakes and broom handles, and so they bent until they broke. Now their jagged joints point to the plums and pears that lie scattered on the ground, rotting, because of my neglect. And I think of Carol's and my promise to shoot each other if we ever got like our mother. I suppose we said it because, deep down, we knew it would never happen to us, knew that even if it did, we could never go through with such a promise. And that this resilience, if it exists at all, is nothing more than the ability to endure.

# ACKNOWLEDGEMENTS

This book would not be were it not for the willingness of my writing partner and husband to go public with the ordeal that is Alzheimer's disease. Tony Wanless wrote openly and honestly about the subject, and encouraged me to do the same. It was tough going at times.

Our thanks to the many people who have helped us along that bumpy road to completion:

Terri Brandmueller for reading and commenting on an early draft of the manuscript; Fiona Tinwei Lam for reading a later version for excerpts; Mary Novik and Jen Sookfong Lee for their wise counsel on some ins and outs of publishing, from contacts to contracts; and all four of these writers for taking energy from their own creative works to offer advice on ours.

Jill Daum for giving thoughtful attention to the sections in our book that make reference to her husband, John Mann.

Nita and Michael Levy of Paul's Club for their kind efforts to help promote this book in its infancy.

John Pearce for his time and consideration in the early days of this project.

Denise Ryan of the Vancouver Sun for the feature article that got publishers looking at *Four Umbrellas*.

The literary press community in Canada for its generosity and enthusiasm, specifically Noelle Allen of Wolsak & Wynn; Deborah Willis of Freehand Books; and Vici Johnstone of Caitlin Press. What a fine circle of support and smarts.

And finally the team at Dundurn Press for outstanding work in bringing our book to literary life during a pandemic: Scott Fraser and Kathryn Lane for sharing our vision and signing us on; Dominic Farrell for his editorial energy; Elena Radic for directing the edits and answering the endless questions; Melissa Kawaguchi for the artful catches; Elham Ali for spreading the word; and Laura Boyle for a cover that so beautifully depicts the storm that was heading our way.

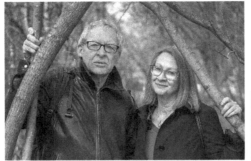

# ABOUT THE AUTHORS

JUNE HUTTON is a teacher and writer who was born and raised in Vancouver. A former northern reporter, she travelled down two Yukon rivers as research for her novel *Underground*, then tapped into her news background for her second novel *Two-Gun & Sun*. June has taught writing to at-risk youths, then to adults in continuing education, and most recently to residents at a treatment centre for addiction. She lives in Vancouver.

TONY WANLESS was born in the Netherlands and raised in Ontario. He worked for several newspapers across Canada, including the *Financial Post* and the *Province*, and blogged for a season for CBC's *The Dragon's Den*. A ghost-writer for business publications, he has always wanted to write his own book, never dreaming this would be it. Tony is taking part in two Alzheimer's studies at UBC Hospital. He lives in Vancouver.